VITAMIN V

A guide to introducing variety into your child's diet (and yours, too!)

Readers are encouraged to go to www.MissionPointPress.com to contact the author or to find information on how to buy this book in bulk at a discounted rate.

MISSION POINT PRESS

Published by Mission Point Press
2554 Chandler Rd.
Traverse City, MI 49696
(231) 421-9513
www.MissionPointPress.com

ISBN: 9781950659302

Library of Congress Control Number: 2019916894

Printed in the United States of America

VITAMIN V

A Guide to Introducing Variety into Your Child's Diet (and Yours, too!)

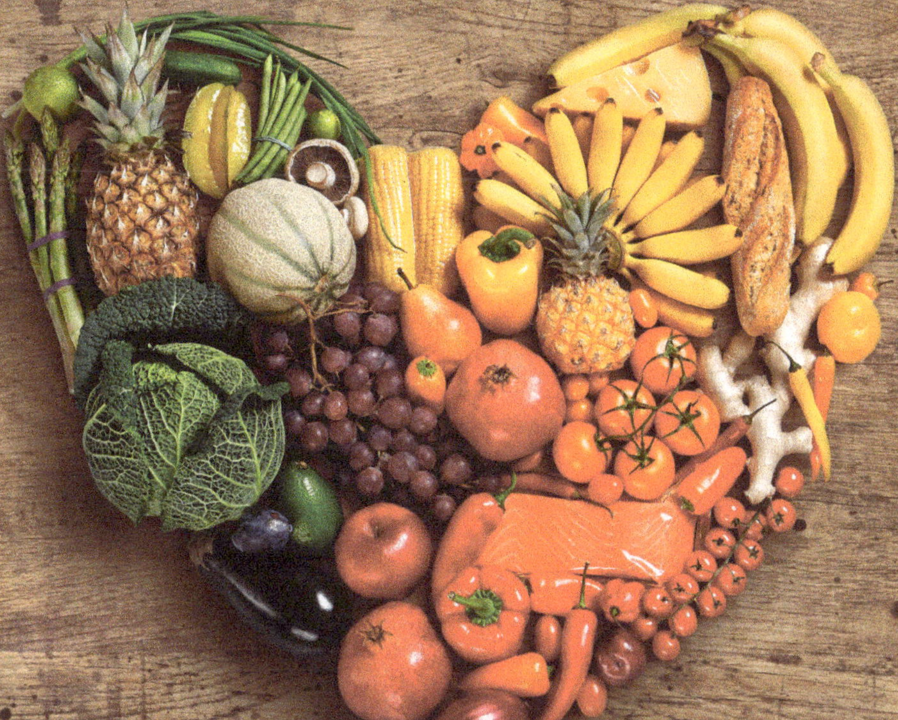

by Natalie Okerson-Sparks M.D.

DEDICATION

I would like to dedicate this book to my father Gary who taught me a solid work ethic, my husband Dean who is my strongest supporter, and my children, Dillon Joseph and Nolan Alexander who inspire me everyday.

TABLE OF CONTENTS

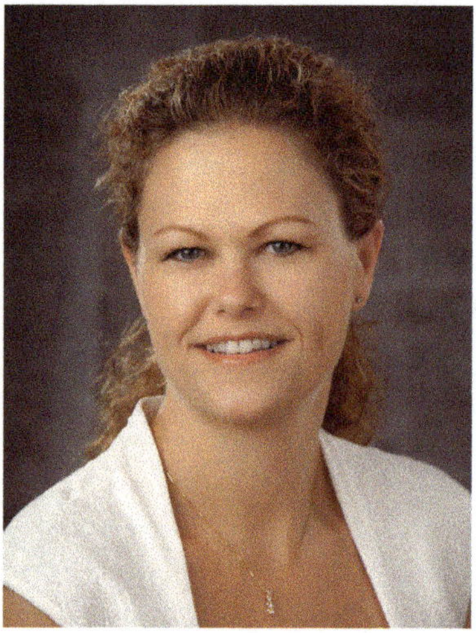

INTRODUCTION

As a family physician, I have counseled many patients on lifestyle modification and dietary recommendations for reasons of preventative medicine, weight loss or maintenance, and chronic disease treatment. I have found that there is a vast array of misinformation all around us, with TV, internet, social media, supplement companies, weight-loss programs, food and beverage corporations, even healthcare practitioners often providing biased information with promising claims and little to no scientific medical evidence to support such claims. This is confusing and misleading for consumers. I have also found that individuals tend to be more successful in implementing changes when they have concrete recommendations on what to do and how to do it.

We are seeing more and more preventable diseases beginning earlier and earlier, even in childhood, directly as a result of what we eat. There is a strong link with our dietary habits and those of our families. As children, we learn directly from those who feed us. Thus it is very important for all caregivers involved to be aware of current dietary recommendations for children. Not only is the concern about what we are consuming *too* much of, but also what we are not consuming *enough* of. I wrote this book with hopes of providing a clear understanding of *WHY* what we eat is so critical to our health and the health of our environment, as well as *HOW* to incorporate what I call the most important dietary factor, "Vitamin V" – VARIETY, into your child's diet and your own. I also felt it important to discuss several topics that often come up in discussions centered on nutrition in the WHAT ABOUT sections.

"Let food be thy medicine and medicine be thy food"
— Hippocrates (often referred to as the Father of Medicine)

Please note that this book is for educational purposes only and not intended to replace regular medical care. Do not discontinue any prescription medications, add or remove supplements, or make drastic changes to you or your child's diet without consulting with your personal health care provider.

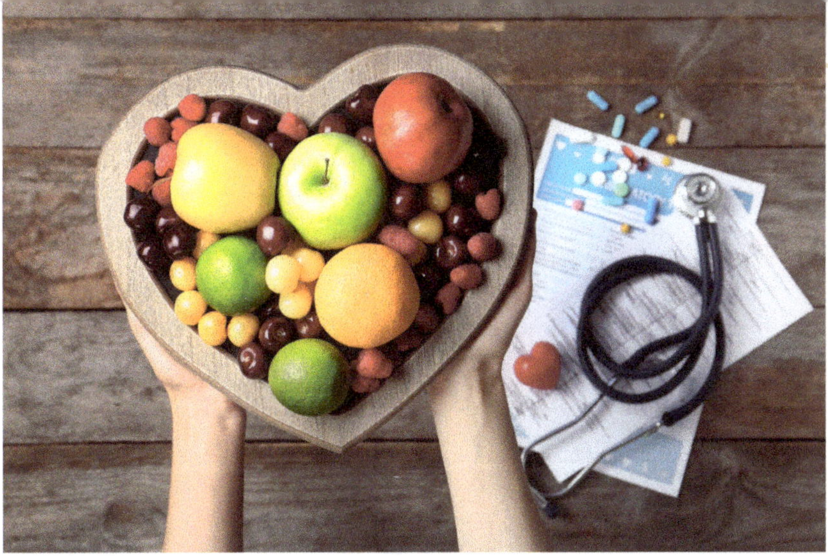

WHY:

DISEASE PREVENTION

There is no argument that certain foods and substances can hurt us. According to the Centers for Disease Control (CDC), in 2016, nearly 65,000 people died in the United States alone from drug overdoses, and this number continues to increase in what is no doubt an epidemic. In the same year, a staggering number of nearly 600,000 people died from cancer in the U.S. But the single deadliest disease, accounting for more than all cancer deaths combined, is heart disease.[1] This includes coronary heart disease (causing heart attacks), as well as congestive heart failure and rhythm abnormalities (which may cause sudden death or stroke, or severe complications from bleeding, due to the treatments needed for such conditions). It has been estimated that about 85.6 *million* Americans are living with some form of cardiovascular disease at any given time, which continues to rise.[2] That is staggering.

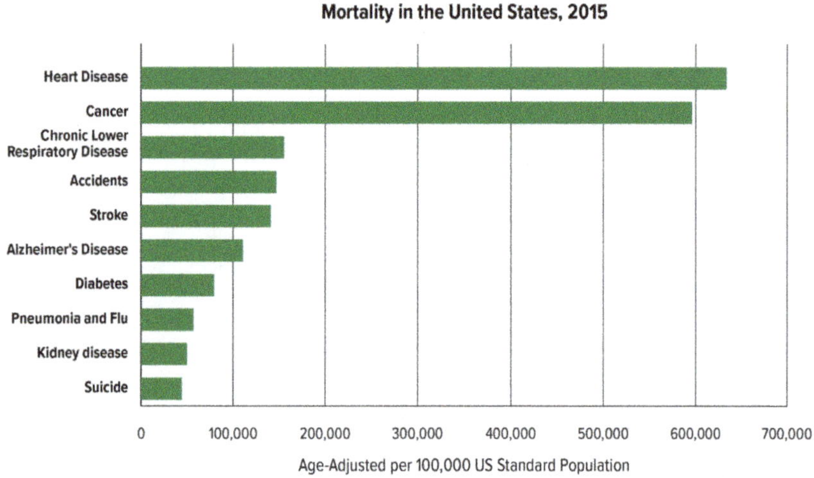

We all strive to steer our kids away from illicit drugs and nicotine, but there is much less attention paid to the potential dangers of what we put in our bodies several times each day, day after day: food. Most people are aware that excess sugar can cause dental decay, weight gain, hyperactivity and worsen diabetes. Most are also aware that fatty fast food is unhealthy and can contribute to high cholesterol, hypertension, obesity and many other conditions. Not to mention the general feeling of being unwell, which is frequently unrecognized due to the tolerant nature our bodies have. But some things aren't as obvious, and I hope to simplify that picture for you in the coming pages.

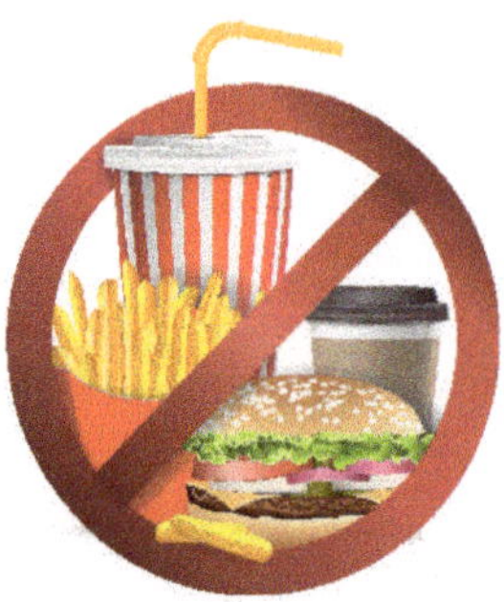

There is a large body of evidence that over time, ingesting pesticides as well as artificial coloring, flavoring and sweeteners, has a detrimental effect on one's health. Does that mean we need to eliminate these things completely from our diet? Well, while that would be ideal, it is neither feasible nor necessary. It is the cumulative ingestion of these items over time that pose a danger. It's a logical conclusion that if we eat more of certain things, we will naturally eat less of others in a compensatory fashion. With that in mind, the primary goal here is increasing a variety of whole foods into our daily diet, and that of our children and in turn reducing or eliminating the consumption of highly processed refined foods.

Furthermore, there are some significant concerns of the excessive amounts of animal products consumed in our country affecting our health. There are so many "diets" existing today it can be not only confusing but overwhelming. Some individuals choose to identify with a label such as vegetarian or vegan for ethical reasons, which should not be discounted. But my intention here is strictly from a health perspective. More recently, we have seen increased use of a label known as a flexitarian, which is a person who consumes mostly plants, but also allows a smaller, less frequent intake of animal products, dairy and/or seafood.[3] My hope is not to define a particular eating style, but rather to educate you about the *WHYs* and *HOWs* of good nutrition, outlining the steps you can take to make healthy dietary choices for yourself and your children and thus helping you to reach your health goals. And ultimately, I truly hope that goal for you and your family is to live better, healthier and longer. Typically, the changes that contribute to successfully reaching that goal will in turn lead to reaching other personal goals, including weight management for adults, for example.

Let's look at some statistics. In many populations around the world, including the United States, several factors have led to an overall shift in eating habits toward animal products and calorie-dense, nutrient-poor, highly processed foods. This shift, as well as other lifestyle and environmental factors, has contributed to a non-communicable disease (NCD) pandemic in countries around the world of every socioeconomic status, not just low-income populations. In recent years, both the United Nations and the World Health Organization have recognized the global threat of NCDs and have attempted to strengthen efforts worldwide to reduce their burden. A study published in *The Lancet* revealed that in 2017, 11 million deaths in 195 countries were attributable to dietary risk factors, including high sodium intake, low intake of whole grains and low intake of fresh produce.[4]

Sometimes our genetic makeup will inevitably lead to a diagnosis of high blood pressure, high cholesterol or other conditions, but our lifestyle choices often accelerate that diagnosis. Conversely, if we choose a healthier lifestyle, we can possibly delay those diagnoses or minimize the number and/or dosages of medications that may be needed to treat the condition.

A Harvard study published in the *Archives of Internal Medicine* tracked 120,000 people in the U.S. over 30 years and found that by swapping beef for a plant protein in one meal per day decreased overall mortality (death from all causes) by 19 percent.[5] According to a study in the journal *Neurology*, a Mediterranean-style diet, which consists of whole grains, healthy plant-based fats, plenty of fruits and vegetables, and less than 3.5 ounces of meat daily (even allowing for a glass of red wine!) showed decreased rates of death from Alzheimer's dementia.[6]

A 2018 article in the journal *American Family Physician* reports the following:

- There is strong evidence that promotes a primary focus on unprocessed foods, fruits and vegetables, plant-based fats and proteins, legumes, whole grains, and nuts.
- Added sugars should be limited to less than 5 percent to 10 percent of daily caloric intake.
- Vegetables (not including potatoes) and fruits should make up one-half of each meal.
- Carbohydrate sources should primarily include beans/legumes, whole grains, fruits, and vegetables.
- An emphasis on monounsaturated fats, such as olive oil, avocados, nuts, and omega-3 fatty acids, such as flax seeds, cold-water fish, and nuts, helps prevent cardiovascular disease, type 2 diabetes, and cognitive decline.[7]

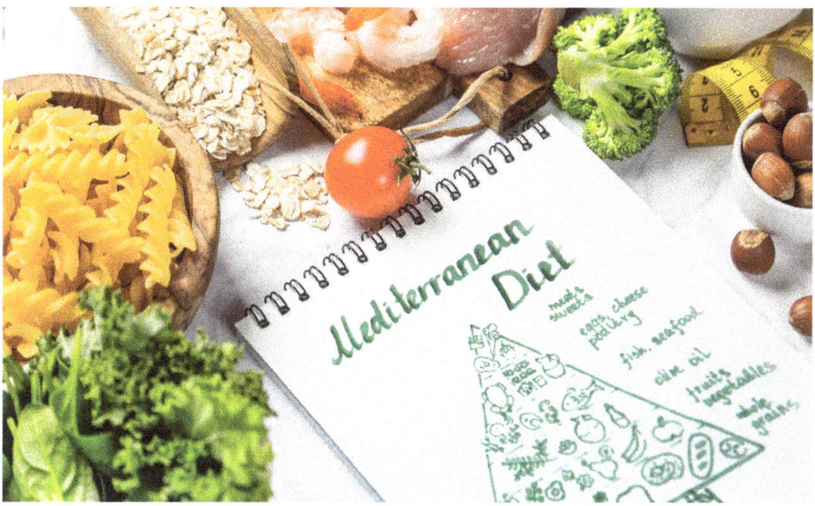

Conversely, consumption of processed meats (bacon, lunch meats, hot dogs) increases the risk of colon cancer by 18 percent, as reported in an article published in *The Lancet Oncology* in 2015[8], and a Harvard study linked a daily serving of two slices of bacon or one hot dog to a risk of early death from heart disease and cancer. This data may prompt one to consider an alternative to sending that lunchmeat sandwich with your child to school on a daily basis.

The goal of consuming a large variety of foods is to obtain adequate amounts of not only macronutrients (proteins, carbohydrates and fats) but also micronutrients (vitamins, minerals, antioxidants and phytochemicals). Why? Because micronutrients have some pretty amazing properties: They have been found to decrease inflammation, hypertension, diabetes, heart disease, cataracts and macular degeneration, as well as aiding in weight loss and decreasing wrinkles and sun damage in the skin. Increased fiber intake – which comes with eating more produce – aids with bowel regularity as well as the lowering of cholesterol and stabilization of blood sugar levels. The Cleveland Clinic reports that individuals who consume plant-based diets have a lower incidence of heart disease, hypertension, diabetes, gastrointestinal disease, colon cancer, breast cancer and obesity.[9] The journal *Progress in Cardiovascular Disease* published an article in 2018 stating that healthy lifestyle choices may reduce the risk of heart attack by over 80 percent, with nutrition playing a key role. Vegetarian dietary patterns reduce cardiovascular disease death and the risk of coronary heart disease (CHD) by 40 percent. Plant-based diets are the *only* dietary pattern to have shown *reversal* of CHD.[10] Wow. Not many medications can make that kind of claim.

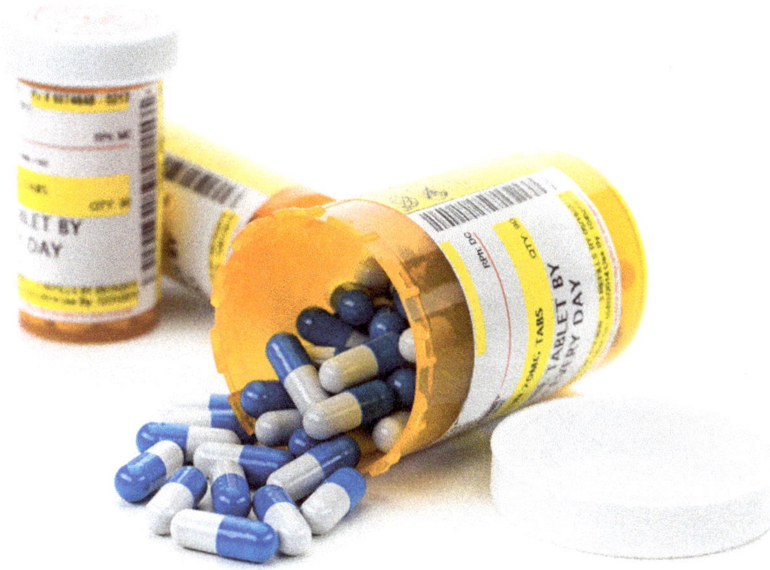

These statistics are reported for adults, so why are we discussing them in a book aimed at nutrition for children? Because research has shown that these diseases are now starting in childhood. And the dietary habits we develop start in childhood. Insulin resistance is a condition that is seen commonly in obese children and adolescents and often leads to type 2 diabetes. The longer patients have diabetes, the higher the potential for complications arising from it. These include:

ATHEROSCLEROSIS (CAD or coronary artery disease): Can cause heart attacks; TIA or transient ischemic attacks, also known as mini-strokes; CVA or cerebral vascular attacks, known as strokes; and PAD or peripheral arterial disease, which at times may lead to extremity amputations (loss of limbs) or the inability to heal severe infections

END-STAGE KIDNEY DISEASE (renal failure): The number-one reason for dialysis (artificial filter for your blood, needed to survive), with a mortality (death) rate of 21 percent two years after diagnosis; also associated with significant morbidity (health risks and complications) due to procedures, infections, anemia and bone loss: significant quality-of-life limitations related to time requirements and cost restraints associated with dialysis

BLINDNESS: The number-one cause of which is diabetes, due to diabetic retinopathy (damage to the blood vessels in the back of the eye), often treatable if diagnosed early

NEUROPATHY (nerve damage): Often leads to persistent numbness and tingling and/or pain in the extremities

GASTROPARESIS (persistent nausea and stomach upset): Caused by slow gastrointestinal movement (otherwise known as stomach and intestines or bowel movement); often associated with neuropathy of the intestines

Trends in child and adolescent overweight

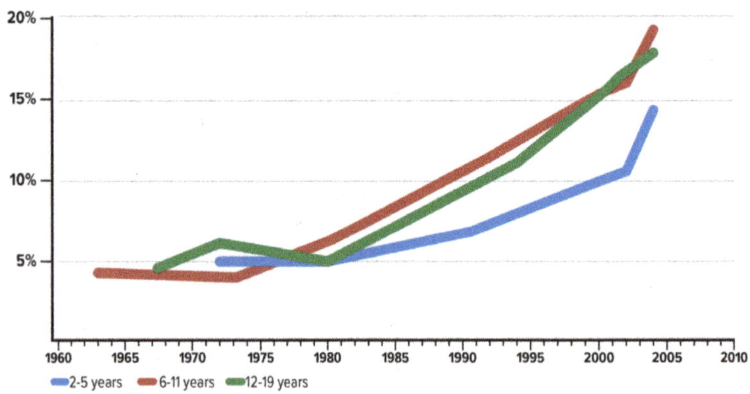

Note: Overweight is defined as BMI >= gender- and weight-specific 95th percentile from the 2000 CDC Growth Charts
Source: National Health Examination Surveys II (ages 6-11) and III (ages 12017), National Health and Nutrition Examination Surveys I, II, III and 1999-2014, NCHS, CDC.

INFECTIONS ANYWHERE IN THE BODY: May be severe and potentially life threatening, due to a weakened immune system and thus poor healing

PRE-DIABETES (or insulin resistance) is seen more and more in younger individuals and has a higher incidence with young girls diagnosed with PCOS (polycystic ovarian syndrome). PCOS is often associated with excess weight and menstrual abnormalities, and can lead to diabetes and potentially fertility issues (difficulty getting pregnant).

The world is getting heavier, and America leads the way

1975—2014 (% of population); Body mass index ≥ 30; Age-standardized

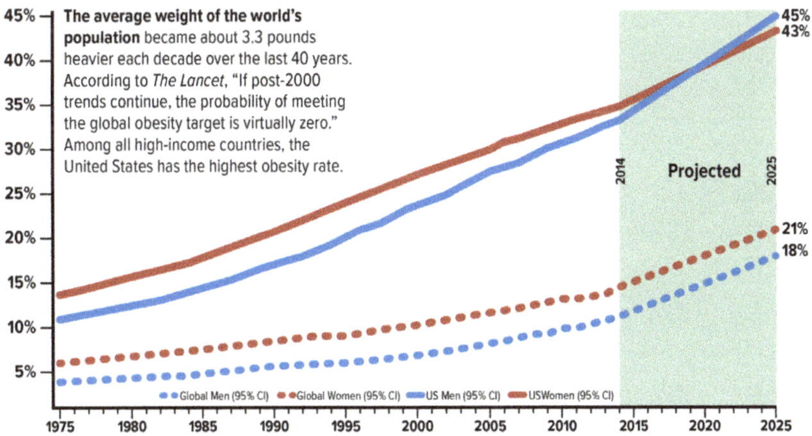

NCD Risk Factor Collaboration (NCD-RisC); Projections: The Lancet 2016; 387:1377-96

We physicians are seeing not only increasing *numbers* of childhood and adolescent obesity but an increase in the *severity* of obesity as well. We are shocked to find atherosclerotic plaques (partial blockages in the arteries) during autopsies of deceased young American adolescents. Of particular significance to note is that this is usually a result of a high intake of animal sterols (mainly cholesterol), which is associated with cardiovascular disease. In the diet, cholesterol is mainly consumed from foods high in animal fat, including meat and dairy products.

As parents we *must* take responsibility for the care of our children, including what they eat. We feed them their first foods and almost everything they consume through school age. We can teach them what is healthy and not healthy for them to eat, so that when they do have the opportunity to decide on their own, we have (hopefully) guided them to make good decisions, just like everything else in life. One thing I would like to emphasize is that it's not only about what to eat *less* of, but also about what to eat *more* of. Increasing fresh plant products and thus decreasing animal products and processed foods, as well as foods with artificial colors, flavors and preservatives, is profoundly significant in our overall health.

On April 1, 2016, the United Nations General Assembly declared the period 2016–2025 as the Decade of Action on Nutrition. Below is a summary of some of the official dietary guidelines developed in certain countries around the world as part of the Food and Agriculture Organization of the United Nations (FAO). These specific countries were selected due to their concomitant recommendations or policies on sustainability, which we will discuss in our next chapter. Published by the FAO and the Food Climate Research Network at the University of Oxford (UK) in *Plates, Pyramids, Planet. Developments in National Healthy and Sustainable Dietary Guidelines: A State of Play Assessment*, they demonstrate many clear commonalities.[11]

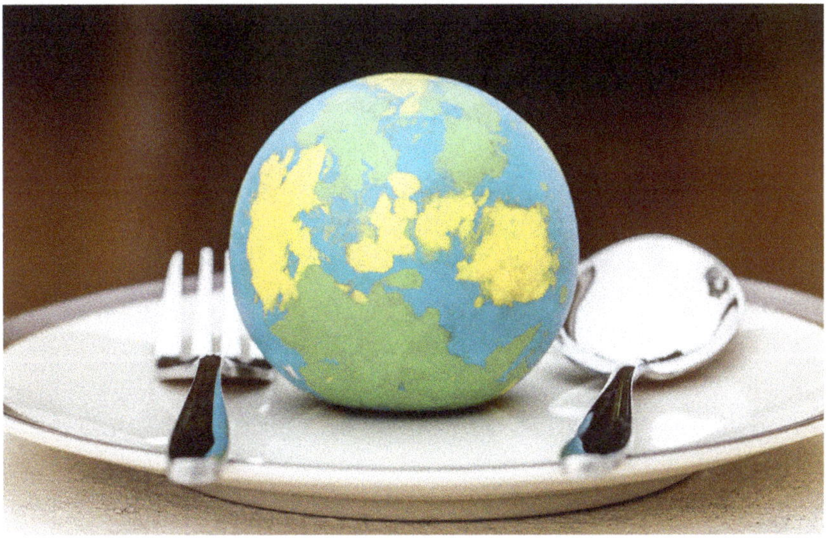

GERMANY: A wholesome diet includes a variable choice, adequate quantities and an appropriate combination of high-nutrient and low-energy food. Choose mainly plant-based foods, which have a health-promoting effect and foster a sustainable diet. Enjoy five portions of fresh, seasonal fruit and vegetables daily, or as often as possible. Include them in each main meal and also as a snack between meals. If cooking them, do it for a short time only. By doing so, you profit by consuming plenty of vitamins, minerals, dietary fiber and phytochemicals and lower your risk of nutrition-related diseases.

BRAZIL: Make natural or minimally processed, plant-based foods the basis of your diet. In addition to the health benefits you will reap for yourself, limiting your consumption of animal proteins will have many related benefits for the environment, including reducing emissions of greenhouse gases responsible for global warming, reducing deforestation caused by the creation of new grazing areas for cattle, and preventing overuse of water. It will also reduce the number of intensive animal production systems, which are particularly harmful to the environment. The crowding of animals, characteristic of these systems, stresses the animals, increases animal wastes, requires systematic use of antimicrobial drugs, pollutes and contaminates groundwater, reservoirs, lakes and rivers, and generates diseases in animals that can be transmitted to humans. These intensive monoculture systems also require production of vast amounts of soybeans and corn for animal feed, the intensive use of water, and a host of chemical pesticides and fertilizers that contaminate sources of water, degrade soil, increase pest resistance and reduce biodiversity.

SWEDEN: Find your way to eating greener, not overeating, and being active! Reducing meat consumption can benefit both your health and the environment. By cutting down on quantity, you may be able to afford to buy meat produced more sustainably, with attention paid to the welfare of the animals. Different animal proteins have different climate impacts: poultry has the smallest impact on climate, followed by pork, while free range-beef and lamb can have other positive environmental effects – animal grazing can help maintain diverse agricultural landscapes and support biodiversity.

QATAR: Emphasize a plant-based diet, including vegetables, fruits, whole grains, legumes, nuts and seeds. When they are available, consume foods that have been produced locally and regionally. Cook and eat homemade food more often, and explore healthy ways to prepare traditional foods.

ESTONIA: Eat in an environmentally conscious way, choosing local, seasonal and traditional foods that are produced sustainably, including plant-based, biologically diverse and species-rich vegetables, fruits, whole grains, legumes, nuts and seeds.

UNITED KINGDOM: Maintain a varied, balanced diet to maintain a healthy body weight. Eat fewer foods high in fat, sugar and salt. Eat more plant-based foods, including at least five portions of fruit and vegetables a day. Value your food - ask about where it comes from and how it is produced, and don't waste it. Choose fish sourced from sustainable stocks, taking seasonality and capture methods into consideration. Moderate your meat consumption, and enjoy more peas, beans, tofu, nuts, and other plant sources of protein. Include milk and dairy products in your diet and/or seek out plant based alternatives. Drink tap water.

FRANCE: Eat a varied diet, including more plant-based foods. Waste less food. Moderate your consumption of meat, both red and white. Buy foods that meet a credible certified standard. And eat fewer foods high in fat, salt and sugar.

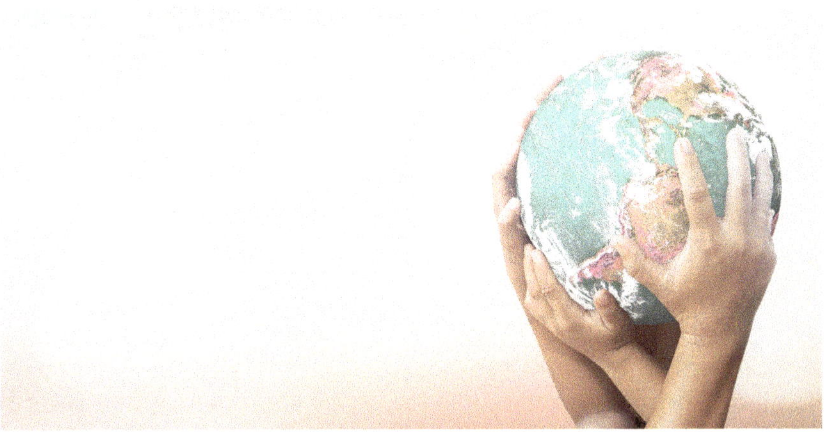

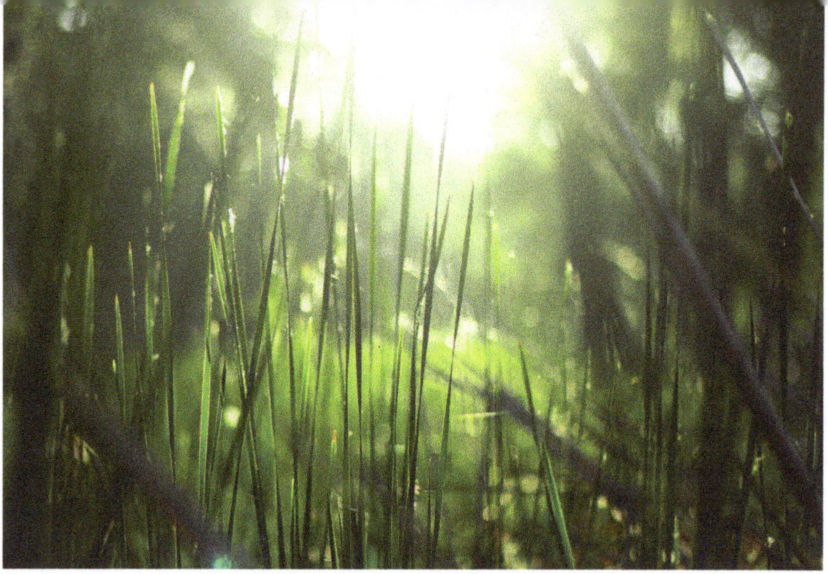

WHY

ENVIRONMENT

Plants are considered a critical resource because of the many ways they support life on Earth. They release oxygen into the atmosphere, absorb carbon dioxide, provide habitat and food for wildlife and humans, and regulate the water cycle. The more demand there is for a variety of plant foods and products, the more their cultivation will benefit our environment. Conversely, there are some significant negative effects we are seeing as a result of the fact that many Americans are over-consuming animal products.

The National Institutes of Health reports that livestock production is responsible for 18 percent of all greenhouse gases. High amounts of energy are required for the feeding, breeding, fertilizers, electricity use and operating costs connected with raising livestock on a commercial scale; therefore, decreasing consumption of animal products would have a beneficial impact on our environment. Each year, the U.S. meat industry creates the same amount of carbon emissions as the entire transportation sector. That includes not only cars, but also public transportation including buses, planes, trains and ships.[12] As a report released from the Food and Agriculture Organization of the United Nations stated: "The livestock sector is a major stressor on many ecosystems and on the planet as a whole. Globally, it is one of the largest sources of greenhouse gases and one of the leading causal factors in the loss of biodiversity, while in developed and emerging countries, it is perhaps the leading source of water pollution."[13]

Elevated greenhouse gas emissions have been associated with respiratory diseases such as asthma, bronchitis and COPD (chronic obstructive pulmonary disease, previously referred to as chronic bronchitis or emphysema), as well as increased infection risk. In November 2017, 15,364 world scientists signed a *Warning to Humanity* calling for, among other things, drastically diminishing our per capita consumption of meat.

Raising animals for human consumption accounts for approximately 40 percent of the total amount of agricultural output in industrialized countries. Land quality decline is associated with overgrazing, as these animals remove much needed nutrients from the soil without the land having time to recover. Deforestation and habitat destruction for the purpose of meat production is contributing to significant biodiversity loss. Nearly 40 percent of the Earth's land surface is being used for livestock farming.

Aquatic ecosystems have also been negatively affected by livestock grazing, which leads to increased levels of phosphates, nitrates, temperature and turbidity, as well as decreased dissolved oxygen and reduced species diversity.[14] The U.S. Environmental Protection Agency estimates that 2,500 gallons of water are required to produce one pound of processed beef. That contrasts with 250 gallons of water needed per pound of soy or 25 gallons needed per pound of wheat. The meat industry causes more water pollution in the U.S. than all other industries combined.[15]

An article published in the *Archives of Internal Medicine* states: "In the United States, livestock production accounts for 55 percent of the erosion process, 37 percent of all pesticides applied, 50 percent of antibiotics consumed, and a third of total discharge of nitrogen and phosphorus into surface water." That is shocking.[15]

Caldwell Esselstyn Jr., MD, is an American surgeon, former Olympic rowing champion and director of the Cleveland Clinic Wellness Institute. His scientific publications number over 150. Thomas Colin Campbell, PhD, is professor emeritus of nutritional biochemistry at Cornell University. Esselstyn and Campbell developed the 2011 documentary *Forks Over Knives*, which demonstrates evidence supporting a plant-based diet in preventing and reversing coronary artery disease as well as strong data on an increased cancer incidence in meat-based diets. The companion to the documentary states environmental statistics as well, including the fact that if the entire U.S. population were to adopt a plant-based diet for just one day, the nation would conserve the following resources:

- 100 billion gallons of drinking water
- 1.5 billion pounds of crops
- 70 million gallons of gasoline
- 33 tons of antibiotics

And the following environmental damage would be prevented:

- 1.2 million tons of carbon dioxide greenhouse emissions
- 3 million tons of soil erosion
- 4.5 million tons of animal waste
- 7 tons of animal emissions

Worldwide, farm animals consume 756 million tons of grain. An equivocal amount would be enough to provide the 1.4 billion people living in poverty around the globe with approximately three pounds of grain per day, twice the amount necessary to survive. Wow, by changing our diet for our own health, we not only help the environment, but also help our world economically and thus save innumerable lives. What a way to impact so much and so many, *and* it costs *less.* The next chapter will pursue this in detail. Albert Einstein summed it up best: "Nothing will benefit human health and increase chances for survival of life on Earth as much as the evolution to a vegetarian diet."[15]

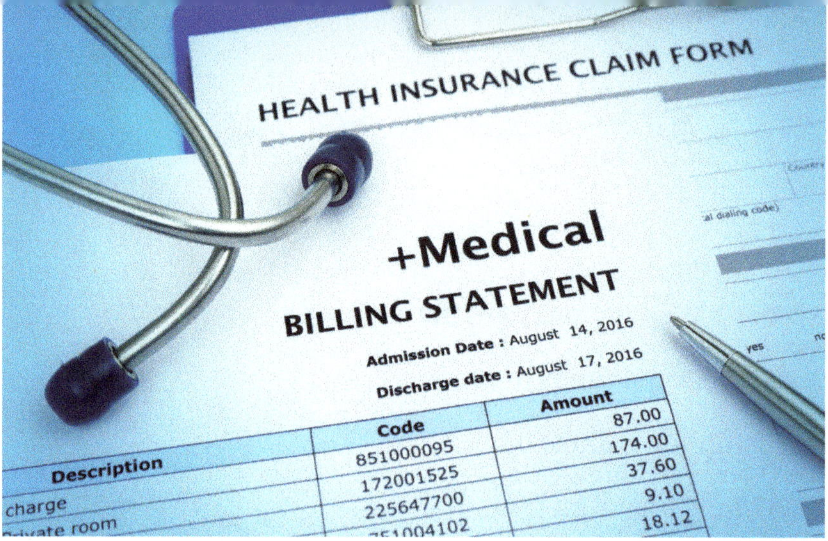

WHY:

COST

The United States has the most expensive healthcare system in the world and some of the least healthy people in the world. Significant dents in both societies and our individual healthcare budgets can be obtained by paying close attention to the foods we eat.

Fruits, vegetables, beans and whole grains generally cost less than highly processed foods, since with the latter, the consumer is also paying for manufacturing and production, as well as research, development, packaging and shipping. If Americans stopped consuming meat at the current recommended guidelines (they currently consume much more than that), it would save $180 billion. Decreasing meat consumption below these levels could save $250 billion and with no meat consumption at all the U.S alone would save between $2-3 trillion.[16]

When it comes to our personal food budgets, we tend to assume that consuming more fresh produce costs more. In contrast, a home-prepared, plant-based diet averages $4-$5 per day vs. $10 per day for a meat-based diet.[17] That said, pre-cut or ready-to-eat fruits and vegetables or small microwavable vegetable packets tend to cost a lot more and have been handled more during the production process, therefore leading to an increased risk of contamination/food poisoning as well as reduced freshness/shelf life. Purchasing the food in whole form and processing it yourself is less expensive, safer and ensures a longer shelf life. And buying produce in season – in smaller quantities to eat right away and/or in larger quantities to can or freeze for consumption year round – also reaps significant cost savings. Local farmers markets are wonderful - support them whenever possible. Produce that needs to be shipped across the country not only decreases the quality due to early picking but also decreases the longevity due to transport time, and on top of that, it costs more.

Even more savings can be achieved by growing your own garden. Starting plants from seed is very affordable and provides your family with large quantities of the freshest seasonal produce possible without concerns about infection from handling. It is also very rewarding and a good life skill to teach your children. They love to participate in not only picking out the seeds, but watering the plants and picking the produce once it is grown and ready to harvest. If you cannot grow a garden due to your living accommodations, consider a community garden or a tower garden, which we will delve into later in the *HOW: FRESH PRODUCE* chapter.

Costs related to food can be secondary - that is, the cost related to the consequences of what we eat. Any number of diseases can be not only prevented, but *reversed*, with a whole-foods, mostly plant-based diet, which cuts down on expensive insurance and medical bills. These costs include extra office visits, urgent care visits, emergency room visits, and diagnostic tests including blood tests and X-rays, as well as more risky high-radiation tests like CT scans. We should also keep in mind the costs and risks associated with medications and their possible side effects.

Many medical conditions are associated with each other, such as hypertension (high blood pressure), high cholesterol and diabetes. Each of these conditions is highly affected by one's diet. As mentioned earlier, in many cases, dietary and lifestyle changes can significantly reduce both the number of medications needed and the dosages of those medications. Most medication side effects are dose dependent, meaning the higher the dose, the more chance there is for a side effect. Medication side effects are vast and are associated with significant morbidity and mortality (sickness and death), and thus potentially unnecessary costs.

In addition, being sick means decreased income as a result of work hours lost, not to mention the immeasurable loss of quality of life, including time spent with family and friends doing enjoyable things with a positive physical, mental and emotional impact. So now that we see why incorporating more "Vitamin V" is smart from a health, environmental and cost standpoint, the next question is *HOW*?

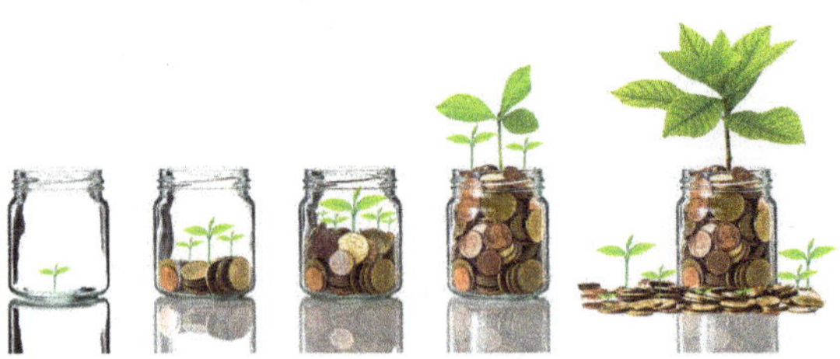

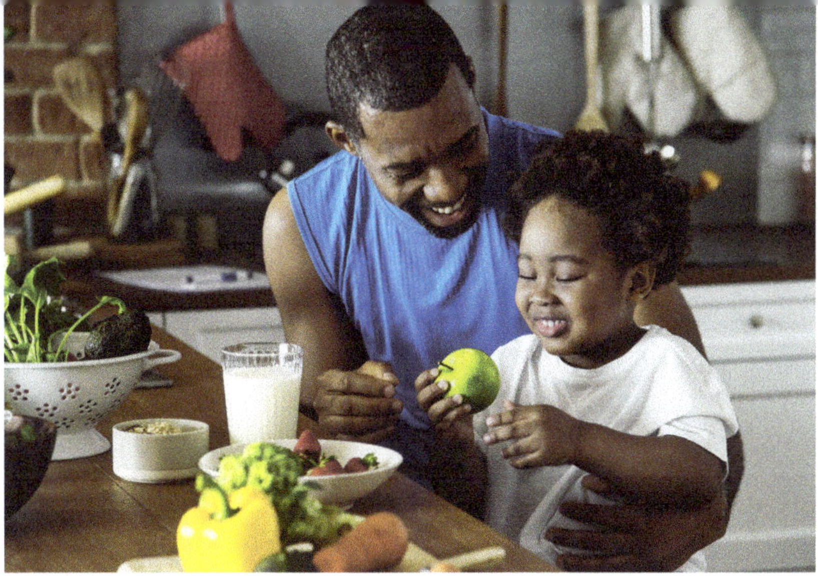

HOW:

GET BACK HOME

Our primary goal as parents is to keep our children safe and healthy, am I right? We expend a lot of effort to protect our children from the dangers of car accidents, house fires, accidental ingestions and second-hand smoke exposure, because we know what devastating consequences those things could have on their health and well being. But far too often, we fail to recognize the potential harm that exists from what we feed them every day. We have become a world of convenience over the last 50 years and have lost the art of cooking in the home due to divided families, dual working parents or single parents, cost restraints, and in some cases pure exhaustion. And at times, let's face it, due to laziness. Many of us easily avoid or minimize the highly identifiable "bad" foods, but we continue to struggle with introducing "good" foods into our children's diet. That's why it is so important to cook at home. This is the only way to know what you and your children are really getting in your meals.

There are endless online resources that offer ideas on how to accomplish this in a faster and/or less expensive manner. To begin with, weekly meal planning is very helpful and actually cuts shopping costs, since we tend to spend less when we stick to a list rather than randomly purchasing items without direction. Prepping food in advance for meals and snacks is another way to save money and control what goes into our family's mouths and bodies. We clearly eat better when we have healthy choices available in front of us. You and your children will be much more likely to eat that donut or bagel if you didn't eat breakfast at home, or to grab that cookie a coworker brought in if you didn't pack some fruit or nuts for a snack. Often, cooking at home produces larger quantities of food, which provides a great opportunity to freeze portions for later use. This is particularly useful for things like spaghetti sauce, soups and healthy breakfast muffins, for example.

Cooking together as a family is a bonding experience and strengthens relationships. Working as a team rather than as competitors, we learn from each other's culinary talents and teach each other. And perhaps even more important, it is focused time, without distractions from TV, computers and cellphones. Having children assist in meal preparation is a valuable life lesson – and frankly, they love to have a role and feel appreciated. Not teaching our children to cook is doing them a huge disservice, both from a nutritional standpoint but from a cost and convenience standpoint as well.

When it comes to introducing a new food, your young child

may need to have it offered eight to ten times before accepting it. So don't be discouraged. Children tend to be more accepting of foods they have helped prepare. Eating dinner as a family on a regular basis has proven benefits for children, including better academic performance, higher self-esteem, a greater sense of resilience, and a lower risk of depression, substance abuse, obesity, eating disorders and teen pregnancy. [*See the reference and recommended reading section for articles detailing and supporting these benefits.*][18, 19, 20]

Not every home-cooked meal needs to be time consuming or multi-course, although those make for special memories indeed. Quick, simple meals with fresh ingredients are far healthier, less expensive, and usually tastier than the restaurant versions of the same thing. Pick any one food item you have on hand and search in cookbooks or online for recipes including that ingredient, which will provide you with several options to consider. Seek vegetarian recipes for greater variety, and feel free to add small amounts of meat or seafood if desired. Try to set a goal of eating out 50 percent less than you currently do - you will find you'll save a lot of money and generally feel better too. Explore new recipes and try to involve your children in this. They may not be receptive at first, but they will surely be proud when their selection is plated for the family! You *can* make it happen, but it does take time to plan, which is completely doable if you make it a priority. And this is something that really should be a priority.

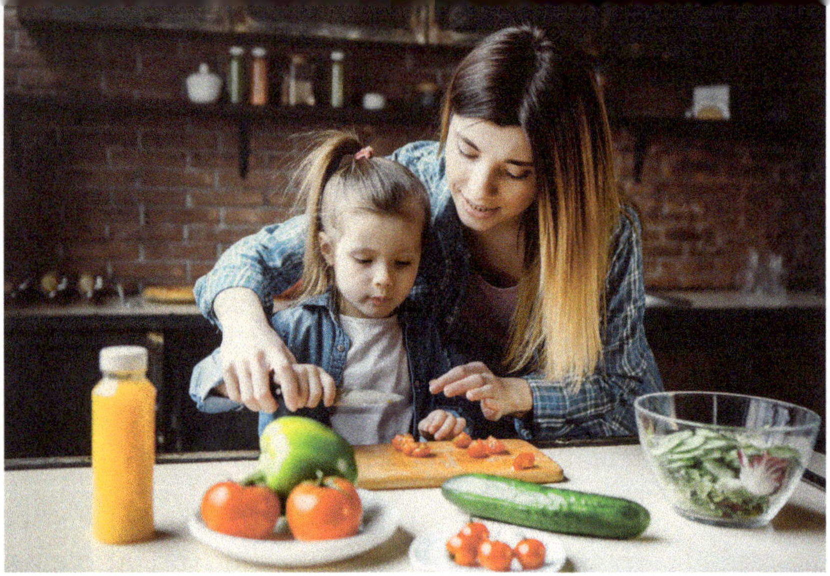

HOW:

INFLUENCE AND TRADITION

There is a natural tendency in American traditions, as well as those of most other nationalities, to use food as a reward or celebration. We all know this. What we need to be cautious about is at what extent we stretch this habit. Too often, these traditions involve foods that are laden with fat and sugar and contain little or no nutritional value. Children's birthday parties and school birthday snacks are prime examples of this. There are so many ways that we can transform these celebrations into activities and events that still include some traditions, but also incorporate foods that are healthier options. And doing so may be accepted by children even more readily than one might expect.

There are also many cases where parents use food (and unhealthy food at that) to "bribe" children. "We will go get ice cream or fast food if you are good for your shots" (immunizations). This is something that I hear all the time in my practice. Each time we do this, children develop an association with these foods in the reward center of their brain. The foods in and of themselves have enough addictive properties – the last thing we need to do is strengthen that association even more psychologically. Rather, discuss what the shots are for and why they are so important.

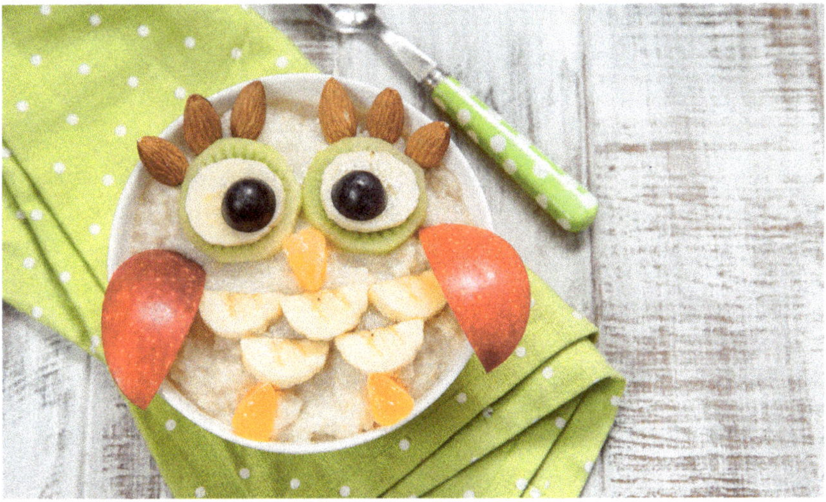

Children are much smarter than we give them credit for. Don't hide from them that something is going to be unpleasant, or they may begin to question you and others. Tell them, (regarding shots) "This *is* going to hurt, but just for a moment, and then we will be done". Reward them with alternate forms of enjoyment, like going to their favorite park or choosing their favorite game to play one-on-one with mom or dad, because what they crave most is time spent with you. Behavioral improvement and encouragement, including potty training, should always be positive. Keeping a chart or calendar with stars or stickers on days your child does well helps him or her to see this objectively. Perhaps end a week full of successes with a choice of a movie for the family or a sleepover with a friend as a reward. Move away from using food, especially sweets, for these events and it will benefit your child significantly in the long run.

Furthermore, we as American families associate food with holiday celebrations. We always have and always will. These foods tend to be rich in fats, sugar and salt and very high in calories - comfort food. Most of us have happy memories of holidays growing up, especially Easter, Thanksgiving, Christmas, and New Year's Eve and Day, and it is for this reason that we find comfort doing or eating the things that remind us of those good times. We naturally want to share these memories and traditions with our families. It is important to continue family traditions, and to have what we eat be impactful from an emotional standpoint, but these foods do not need to be laden with fat, sugar and salt. Changing the face of comfort foods has a lasting impact. Create new traditions.

Recognizing that not only can foods harm us, but that food can also heal us, is something many are unaware of. I believe we fail to recognize the powerful influence we have on our children. This parental influence will impact and form the choices your children will make for the rest of their lives and further impact their contacts whom they influence. Recognizing this brings on a new sense of importance into all the decisions we make, not only with regard to the foods we buy and where we buy them, if and how we grow them, and how we prepare them, but also with regard to how we eat them-with other people, especially with our family. The communal gathering during meals is a time of bonding, and it can be very therapeutic. Encourage your child to seek out another child sitting alone at mealtime in school - friendliness is happiness.

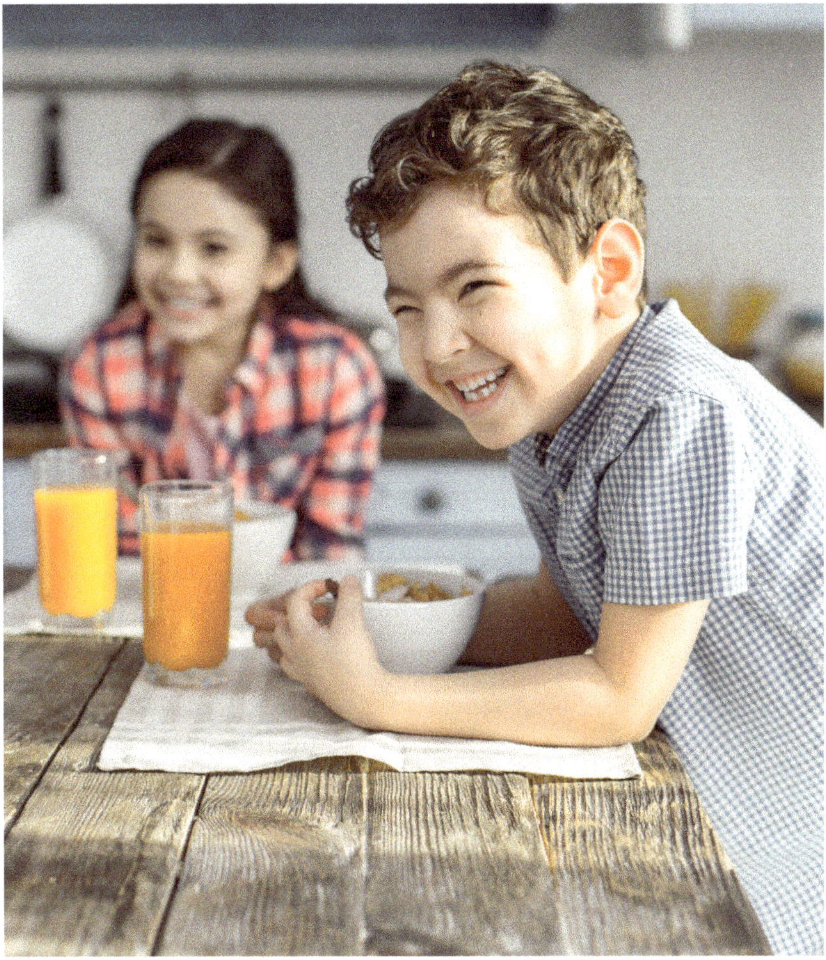

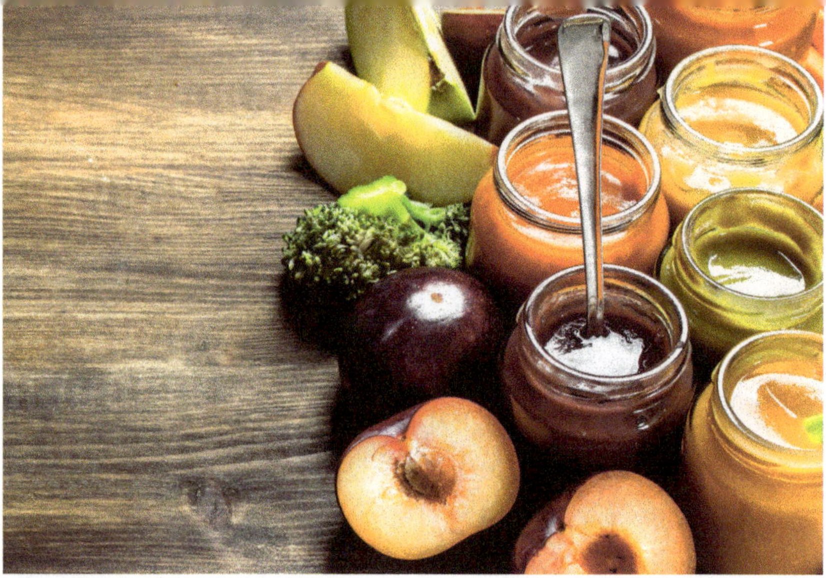

HOW:

THE EARLIER THE BETTER

The best advice I can give you for instilling in your child the importance of healthy eating habits is to start early! If a mother hasn't already begun doing this during her pregnancy, then she should start as soon as her baby is born. Clearly, breast milk is best. For those unable to breastfeed or for those who choose not to, current formulas are very safe and complete. Mothers should consume the most nutritious foods possible not only during pregnancy, but while breastfeeding as well. Obtaining adequate amounts of water is especially important, but so is getting a wide variety of whole foods and the vital nutrients these provide.

There has been more and more evidence as of late that earlier introduction to a variety of foods (4-6 months of age) *decreases* the incidence of allergies and some food intolerances and is associated with healthy brain development.[21] It is also evident that with early introduction of first foods, the more accepting children seem to be. However, if your family has a history of severe allergic reactions to food, please seek the advice of your child's doctor before the introduction process. Making your baby's food at home is easy and much more affordable than buying commercially produced items from a store. One would be amazed at how far a single sweet potato can go! Also, the variety of baby foods available in stores are limited (although increasing rapidly).

When introducing first foods, the key is to stick to individual foods and offer them as a very smooth puree. Identification of allergies requires foods being introduced one at a time. Also, allergic reactions typically do not occur with the first exposure to a food, so it is recommended to use the same food for several days before moving on to the next. Reactions in babies can include a variety of symptoms and signs, including fussiness, rash, vomiting, difficulty breathing, and changes in the stool, among others. Contact your health care provider if your child develops any of these reactions.

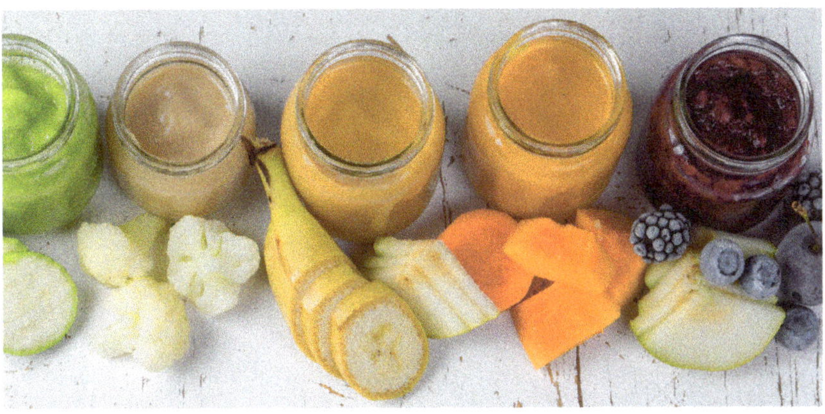

Once all first foods have been introduced, combinations can

be given. Peel and chop vegetables or fruits into smaller chunks, steam until soft, and then blend them with purified water to a smooth consistency. When the mixture has cooled completely, it can then be packaged into small containers and refrigerated or frozen for later use. Softer foods do not need to be steamed and should preferably be processed raw. Many more items can be given in this way than are available in store-bought baby foods. Be sure to wash all produce well just prior to processing and use organic whenever possible.

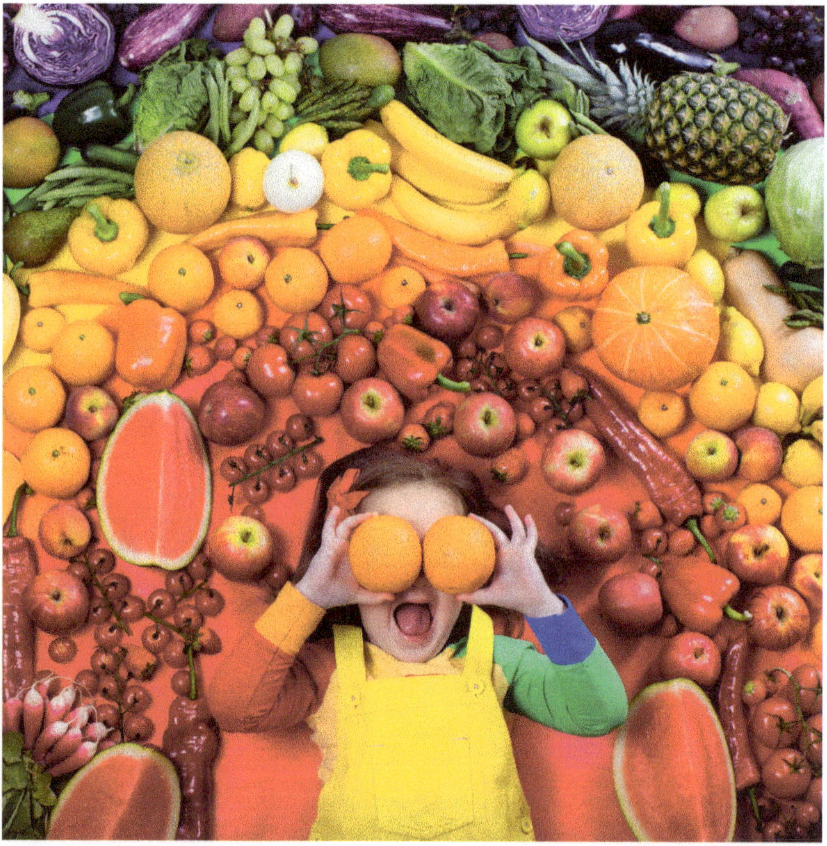

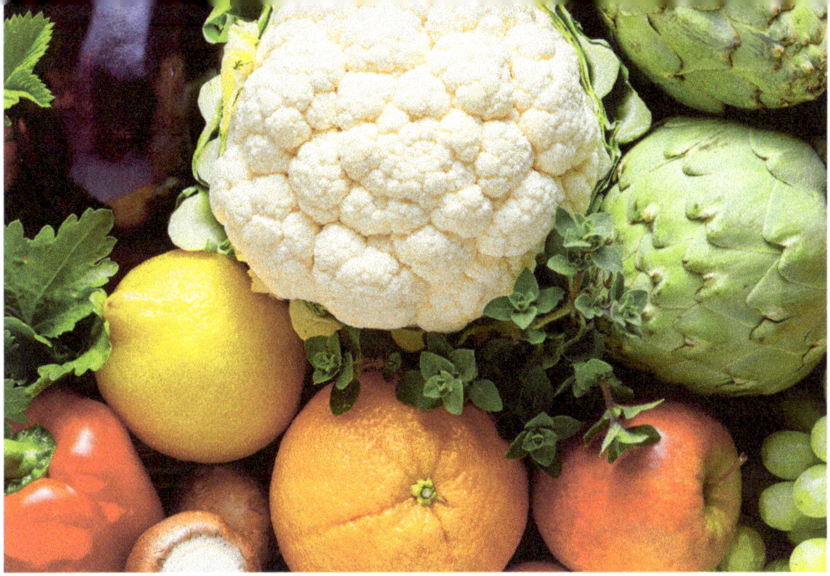

HOW:

VARIETY, HEART AND SOUL

I recommend trying produce in a variety of different ways. If it isn't accepted raw, try it steamed. Or grilled, baked, in a soup, in a pureed sauce, mixed with other favorite foods, or combined with a different spice/herb. Often we hear that kids are not fond of Brussels sprouts. Part of this may be due to how it is prepared. If it is frozen and reheated, it tends to be water logged and not palatable. But if it is fresh and steamed or roasted (even with a little pure maple syrup on it), it tends to be tolerated much better. Alternately, using raw Brussels sprouts to make a slaw can be a brand-new way of trying them with a completely different taste. Or maybe we need a break and should reintroduce it again in another six months. Never stop trying!

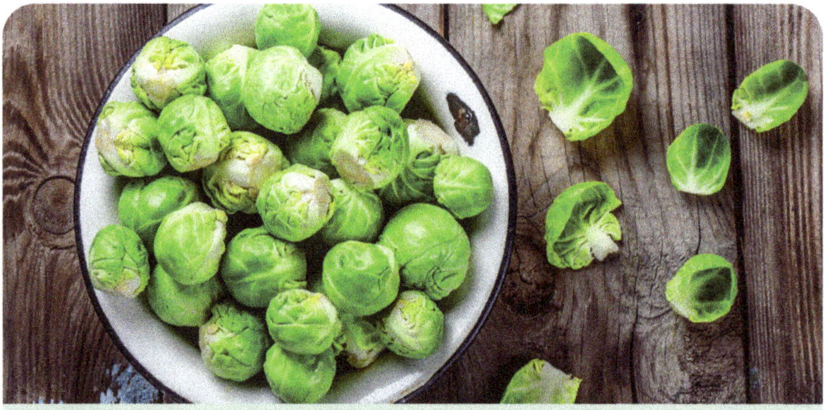

Shredded Brussels Sprouts Salad

Serves 4-6

- 12 oz fresh Brussels sprouts, sliced thinly, cores discarded
- ¼ c dried cranberries
- ¼ c chopped pecans
- 1 raw pear, chopped

Maple-Balsamic Vinaigrette

- 2 tbsp EVOO
- 2 tbsp balsamic vinegar
- 1 tbsp pure maple syrup
- 1 tsp Dijon mustard
- salt and pepper to taste

Add sliced sprouts to a large bowl and mix with cranberries, pecans and pear. Mix dressing ingredients in a jar and shake to combine. Pour vinaigrette over salad and serve. You may also add crumbled gorgonzola/blue cheese if desired.

I find that some foods are more readily accepted if we incorporate them into an already favorite food. For example, if your child loves macaroni and cheese - and who doesn't? You have many possible options:

Try using alternative pastas/noodles. There are several to choose from, including not only different grains (including gluten-free), but also different plant-based proteins like lentils and garbanzo beans, Some of these latter "protein-plus" options are free of the coarse texture that may make other whole-grain pasta varieties less palatable to children.

Add a favorite blanched or steamed vegetable, such as peas, broccoli, cauliflower, carrots or green beans. Shelled edamame (soy beans) would also be a good choice.

Add a teaspoon of nutritional yeast (not regular yeast), which adds B vitamins and is a complete protein with a nutty taste that kids won't even notice in small amounts. It can also be added to popcorn - often undetected - for extra nutritional benefit.

Another way to introduce variety is to vary the grains of crackers you purchase - there are many options to choose from, such as whole wheat, multigrain, multi-seed, lentil and others. Crackers go great with hummus, and many kids (and adults) love hummus. It no longer needs to be made simply from garbanzo beans (chickpeas), and it is affordable and easy to do at home. You can also use canned, drained white beans or black beans, shelled edamame (soybeans) or even cooked sweet potatoes. You can alter the spices to your liking and leave out the traditional tahini (ground sesame seed paste) if you prefer. Making hummus at home also allows for less oil and salt than is typically used in store-bought varieties. And it's inexpensive!

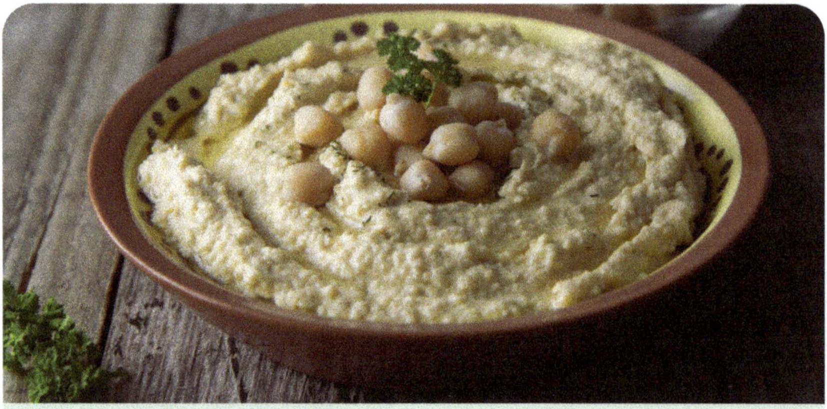

Traditional Hummus

Serves 8-10

- (2) 15-oz cans chickpeas/garbanzo beans, drained and rinsed (or substitute an equal amount of cannellini beans)
- ¼ c tahini
- ¼ c fresh squeezed lemon juice
- ¼ c cold water, more or less, as needed
- 1-2 medium cloves garlic, chopped
- ½ tsp ground cumin
- 1 tsp salt
- EVOO to drizzle on top, if desired

Blend all ingredients in a food processor or blender for about one minute, or until smooth. Serve with crackers, pita bread or raw vegetables. If you love basil, you could add one or two tablespoons of prepared pesto for a different version of this hummus. Or blend in a roasted red bell pepper, which you can either purchase or roast yourself. Using ¼ -½ of the pepper would be adequate depending on your preference. Typically less with kiddos.

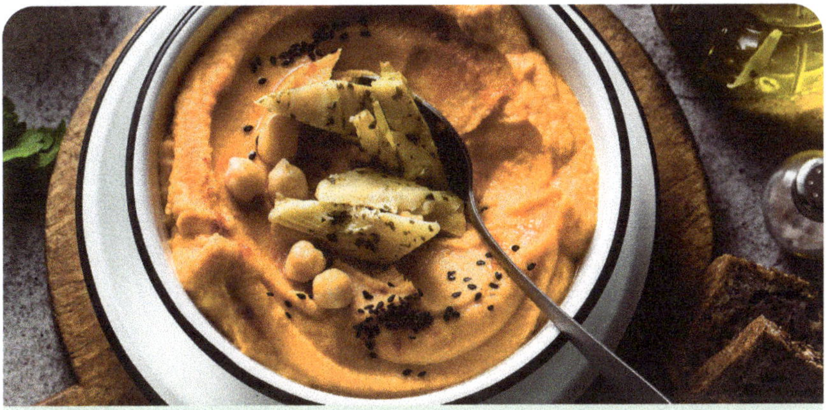

Sweet Potato Hummus

Serves 8-10

- 1 small sweet potato (or ½ large), baked or roasted
- (1) 15-oz can chickpeas, drained and rinsed
- juice of ½ lemon
- ¼ c tahini (optional)
- 2 tbsp avocado or other neutral flavor oil
- ½ tsp salt
- ½ c water or more if needed

After allowing potato to cool, remove the flesh from the skin and mix all ingredients in a food processor or blender for about a minute to desired consistency. You could add some cinnamon as well if desired

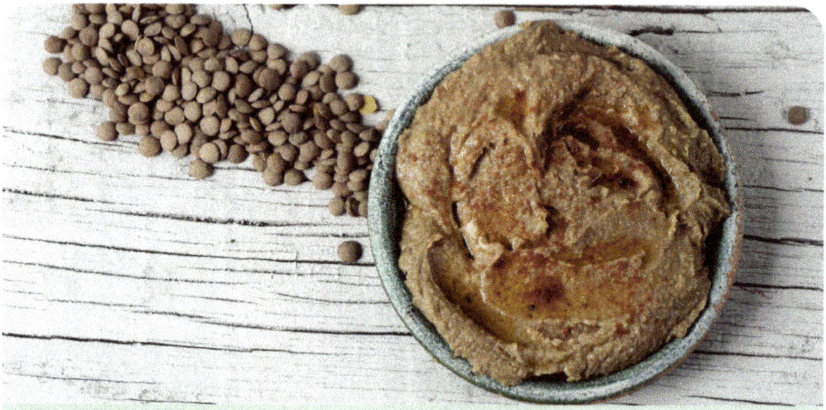

Lentil Hummus

Serves 8

- 1 c yellow lentils, uncooked
- 2 c water
- 1 tsp salt
- ½ c fresh cilantro, chopped
- 3 tbsp tahini (optional)
- 2 tbsp EVOO
- 1-2 cloves garlic, chopped
- juice from ½ lime
- 1¼ tsp cumin
- ¼-½ tsp cayenne, if desired, for extra spice

Bring water and lentils to boil. Reduce heat to medium-low and cook until the lentils are soft and the water has been absorbed, about 40 minutes. After cooling, mix all ingredients in a food processor or blender until smooth. You can use the same recipe and replace the lentils with a can of drained black beans. The tahini can be omitted if you don't have it on hand or prefer not to use it. You can also blend in a seeded and chopped jalapeno if you like extra spiciness.

Yogurt is a common snack food with nutritional benefits that come in an array of varieties that I recommend trying. If you use traditional cow's milk-based yogurt, try to purchase organic Greek, French or Icelandic options, but also consider adding a coconut milk-based yogurt, a soy-based brand, and/or an almond milk brand to your grocery cart. The most important consideration with *all* yogurt varieties is to watch the sugar content. Therefore it is best to purchase the plain flavor (without sugar) and add your own fruit and honey, pure maple syrup or dates for sweetness if desired. Kids always like special things made just for them, and yogurt parfaits usually go over very well. Layer yogurt with fruit and/or granola in a clear glass and voila, easy!

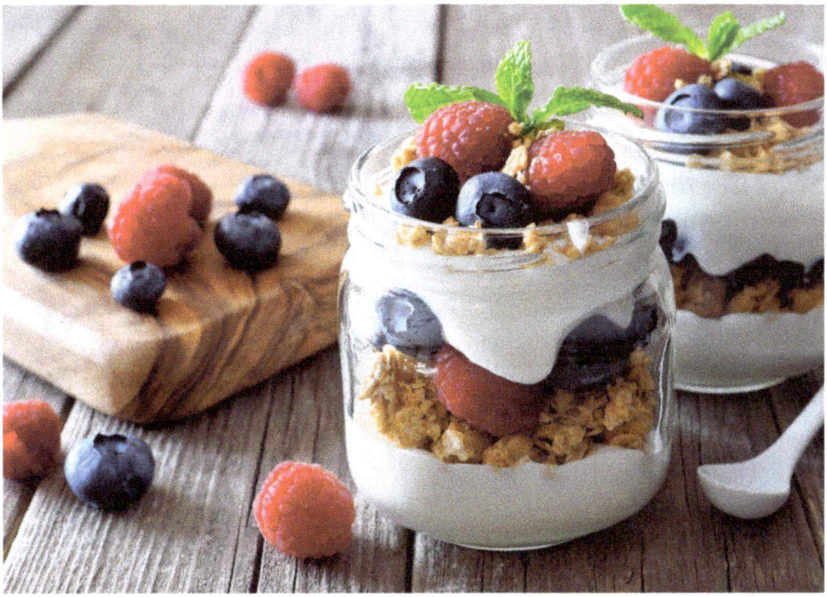

Varying the oil you use to prepare meals is a good idea, too. Some are better for cooking, and some better for dressings or finishing. Generally speaking, it is best to use unrefined oils, but you do need to be aware of the smoke point of each oil when cooking with it (the temperature at which the oil burns and visibly smokes). Canola, peanut and vegetable oils are chemically processed, so try to avoid these. Palm oil is used in massive amounts in processed foods, especially snack foods and condiments. Palm oil produces 38 percent of the world's total vegetable oil supply, and it is reported that each human consumed an average 17 pounds of palm oil per person in 2015.[22] The palm industry has been criticized for negative impacts on the natural environment, including deforestation, loss of natural habitats and threatened endangered species - yet another reason to limit it in your cooking.

Extra-virgin olive oil (EVOO) has heart-healthy monounsaturated fats but a low smoke point, so it is better used for sautéing and drizzling rather than roasting or frying (better to avoid frying anyway, due to the absorption of the oil into the food and thus dramatic increases in fat and calorie intake). Avocado oil is great to cook with, as it has a neutral flavor and high smoke point. Coconut oil is high in saturated fats, which you want to limit in quantity, but in its unrefined form it has a wonderful coconut taste which adds great flavor to raw desserts and in small amounts to air-popped popcorn as a substitute for butter. However, it has a very low smoke point, so you need to watch that if you are cooking with it. The refined version of coconut oil is more forgivable with heat, but unflavored. Safflower oil is low in saturated fats, has a very high smoke point, and is best purchased in the cold-pressed version. Sesame oil has a wonderful but strong flavor, so a little goes a long way. It is particularly good in stir-fry dishes.

Flaxseed oil is high in omega-3 fatty acids, but you can't cook with it. It oxidizes rapidly, so the beneficial qualities do not last very long. It is difficult to obtain the nutrients from flaxseeds when consuming them whole, so the best way to get the most bang for your buck is to grind them yourself right when you need them. (In large quantities or with other grains may use a blender, or in small quantities use a mortar and pestle or a spice grinder). They are wonderful to add to muffins, cookies, pancakes, flatbreads, waffles and granolas, and they are also good in raw treats. They contain many nutritious qualities, including high fiber, which aids with satiety (keeping us feeling full), promotes bowel health (we all want that!), lowers cholesterol, and helps regulate steady blood sugar levels. It is important to note, though, that flax seeds need to be stored in a cool, dark place, such as your freezer, which - as with other seeds, nuts and flours - will lengthen its shelf life.

In baking, you can often substitute alternative flours in many recipes for more variety. Be sure to review recipes when doing this, as some (particularly coconut flour) may have a much higher fiber content, and thus the amount needed in a recipe may be substantially less than with white flour. I often use whole oats blended to a powder for half of the flour recipe, or almond flour. My kids do not like the texture of quinoa, so I often use quinoa flour in our pancakes. Garbanzo bean flour makes some great flatbreads that you can serve with hummus or chutneys, or as a gluten-free pizza dough. Even fermented lentils and rice can be used to make small soft tortillas with various delicious filling options. Teff flour, with its nutty taste, is great in molasses or peanut butter cookies. It is also the main ingredient used in Injera bread, a staple in Ethiopian cuisine. I've yet to master that one. Teff is the smallest whole grain in the world and is high in protein and fiber. As mentioned earlier, keeping your flours and nuts stored in the freezer will preserve them much longer, and they do not freeze, so you don't have to worry about thawing.

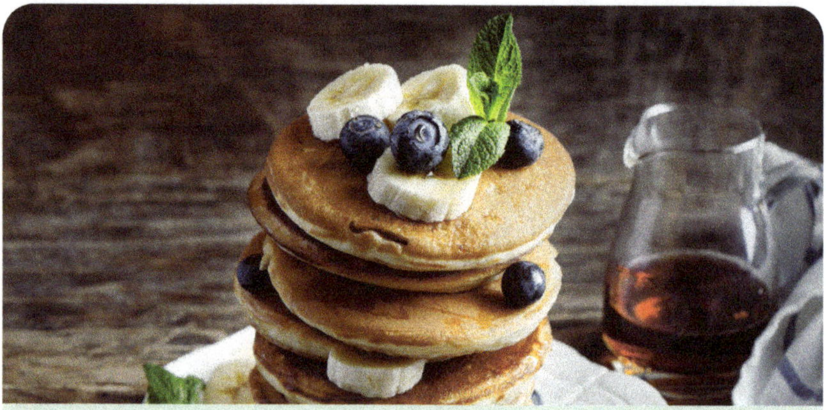

Quinoa Flour Banana Pancakes

Makes 6 pancakes

- ½ c quinoa flour
- ½ c unbleached all purpose flour
- 1 tbsp sugar
- 2 tsp baking powder
- 1 tsp cinnamon
- ¼ tsp salt
- 1 very ripe banana, mashed
- ¾ c milk of choice, dairy or non-dairy
- 1 egg or chia egg
- 1 tsp pure vanilla extract

Mix the dry ingredients in a large bowl. In a separate bowl, whisk the wet ingredients with the mashed banana. Add wet ingredients to dry ingredients and stir well - the batter will have some lumps from the banana. Heat a griddle to 325 degrees F and spray with cooking spray. Pour ¼ c batter portions onto the griddle; flip once the bubbles have broken on the surface and the edges start to dry and continue to cook another couple minutes until done.

Note: I sometimes like to add blueberries to the batter. Serve with warmed real maple syrup.

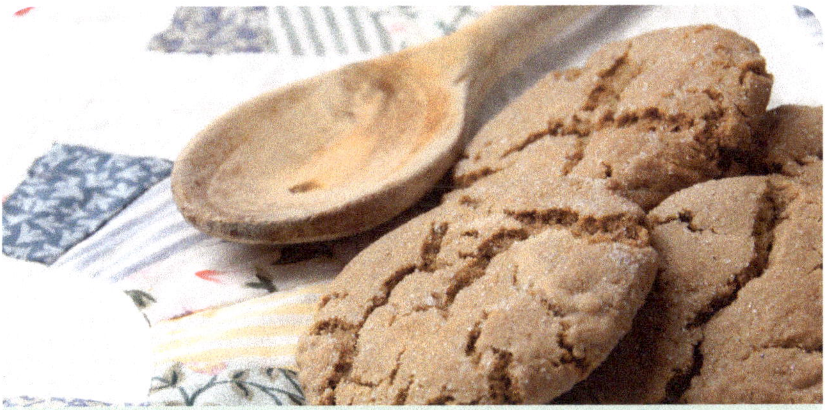

Teff Molasses Cookies

Makes about 16 cookies

- ½ c plus 2 tbsp teff flour
- ¼ c refined coconut oil (not melted)
- ¼ c maple syrup
- ¼ c molasses
- 3 tbsp pumpkin puree
- 1 tsp ground cinnamon
- ¼ tsp ground allspice

- ¼ tsp salt
- ½ tsp baking soda

Heat oven to 350 degrees. Line a baking sheet with parchment paper. Cream together the coconut oil and pumpkin with a wooden spoon, then add in the molasses and maple syrup. In another bowl stir the teff flour, spices, baking soda and salt. Add wet ingredients to dry and stir well. Refrigerate the dough for 10-15 minutes. Drop dough by heaping tablespoons onto a cookie sheet and bake for approximately 18-20 minutes. Allow to cool completely before enjoying.

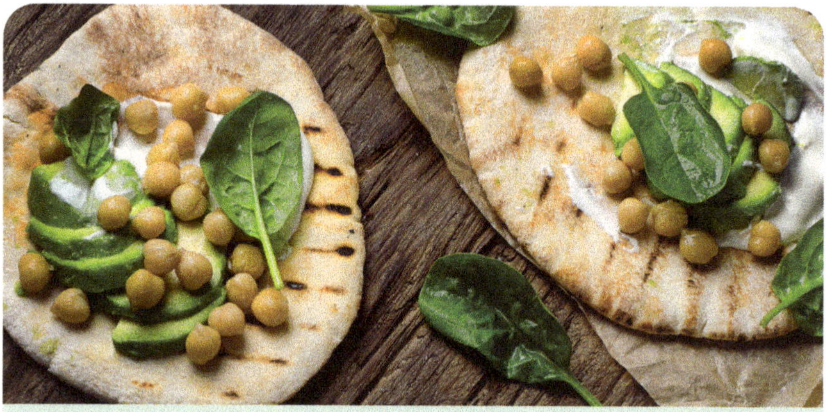

Chickpea Flatbread

Makes 4 flatbreads

- 1 c chickpea flour (available in health food stores or large grocery chains)
- 1 c plus 2 tbsp water
- ¾ tsp salt
- ¼ tsp cumin
- 1½ tbsp EVOO, plus more for brushing the skillet and the finished

flatbread (I like to use garlic infused olive oil for this recipe)

Whisk together the flour, water, salt, cumin and 1½ tbsp EVOO. Allow to rest, covered, at room temperature for 2-3 hours. When ready to cook, preheat the broiler to high with a small 6" cast iron skillet (be sure to always use an oven mitt when handling the hot skillet). Stir the batter again. When the skillet is hot, carefully brush it with olive oil and pour in a thin layer of batter. Cook under the broiler until the flatbread has firmed and browned, about 4-5 minutes. After removing it from the pan, brush the pan with more olive oil and cook the remaining flatbreads. Cut each into triangles after cooling and serve plain or with a topping/dip of your choice. These are not intended to be used as wraps. They can also be cooked on a stovetop over med-high heat once the pan is preheated but would need to be flipped midway.

For those who consume rice, try replacing white rice (which is stripped of its outer layers, fiber and beneficial nutrients) with brown rice, wild rice, red rice or better yet, black rice. Black rice has the highest amount of antioxidants, protein and fiber of all rice varieties and is a good source of iron. Black rice is also known as forbidden rice. Thousands of years ago in ancient China, Chinese noblemen banned its consumption among anyone who was not royal or of the highest elite class.

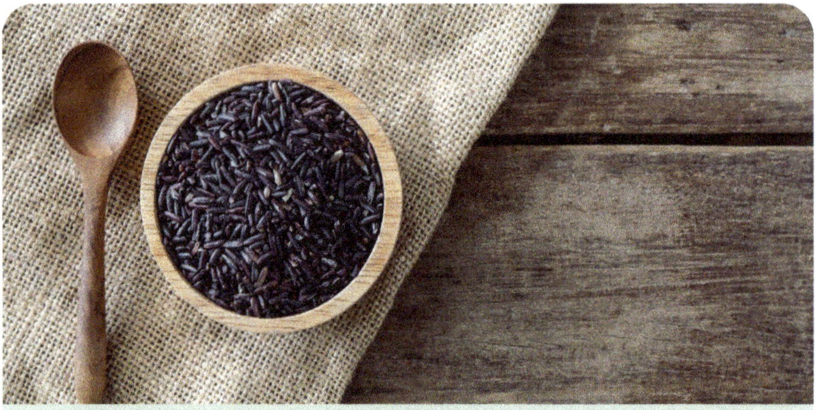

Black Rice with Ginger and Lime

Makes 2-3 servings

- 1 tbsp unrefined coconut oil
- 1 tbsp finely minced ginger
- ¾ tsp salt
- ½ c black rice
- 1 c water
- juice of ¼ lime
- top with chopped cilantro for garnish (optional)

Heat coconut oil on medium-low heat and saute ginger until fragrant. Add salt and rice and stir well. Add water, bring to a simmer, cover, and cook for approximately 40 minutes, or until the rice is soft and water absorbed. Let rest 5 minutes, then fluff rice, squeeze in the lime juice, and serve. Hmmm, I bet black beans and black rice would go together quite well too. Perhaps with a southern American flare. Maybe experiment with that next!

There have been valid concerns about arsenic found in high amounts in rice products. Arsenic has been labeled a human carcinogen (linked with causing cancer), especially inorganic arsenic found in soil from pesticides and irrigation water. Rice is particularly susceptible due to its growing conditions - it absorbs more arsenic than other food crops.[23, 52] Organic rice from California, India or Pakistan has the least arsenic vs. non-organic rice grown in Arkansas, Texas, Louisiana and most other U.S. states, according to a *U.S. Consumers Reports* study of 223 samples of rice products. One way to reduce arsenic in rice by 40-60 percent is to cook it in excess water (6-10 parts water to one part rice). It is also beneficial to rinse the rice or even soak it for 48 hours before cooking, pouring off the water and rinsing every 8-12 hours, similar to soaking beans. When the rice is done cooking, drain off the excess water. Unfortunately, the rinsing process can also wash away many of the nutrients.[24]

Having variety in our diet has the advantage of providing the various nutrients we need in our diet, as well as diluting or minimizing the inevitable toxins or carcinogens we may be exposed to despite our best efforts. The more we "put all our eggs in one basket," so to speak, when it comes to our food choices, the more we risk ingesting larger quantities of unwanted chemicals and substances. Pulling in the variety of good and diluting out the bad is one way to think of it.

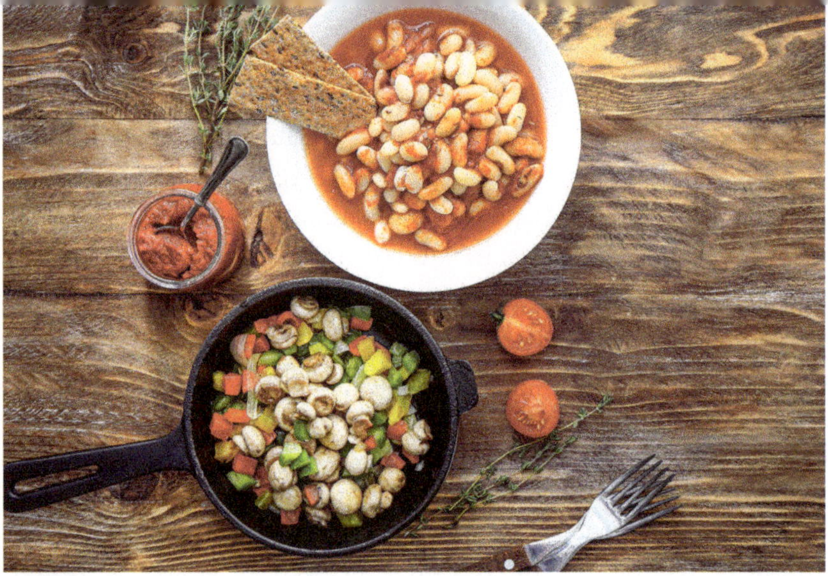

HOW:

"HEALTHIFY" RECIPES

Other avenues of adapting recipes to the palate of various members of your family while adding even more nutritional value is something I call "healthifying." For example, traditional chicken noodle soup typically contains chicken, celery, carrots, onions, broth and noodles. In addition to those, I recommend adding a variety of other ingredients, such as fresh fennel bulb (chopped and sautéed with onions as well as garlic - always add garlic!), great northern beans (canned and drained, or dried and precooked), and/or parsnips. You could also add chopped kale or spinach in the last 20 minutes of cooking. Any or all of these additions could be used or substituted to the taste of the individual or family. Another recipe that can easily be "healthified" is a favorite of many families - chili. Adding finely chopped bell peppers, mushrooms, onions, summer squash, zucchini, eggplant, carrots, and so many more vegetable varieties can make it not only more healthy but more interesting. When cooked down and combined with beans, tomato sauce, and traditional spices for chili, these additions are usually very well received.

You can do the same with spaghetti sauce. Use a variety of fresh vegetables and cook them down with stewed tomatoes, tomato sauce, and fresh or dried basil and parsley. Puree with an emulsion blender. This eliminates the texture issue many kids have. It has been a huge success in our family - not only for the children, but for many picky adult guests as well! This sauce, served with higher-protein pasta and a side salad, is a hearty and healthy meal for any growing child.

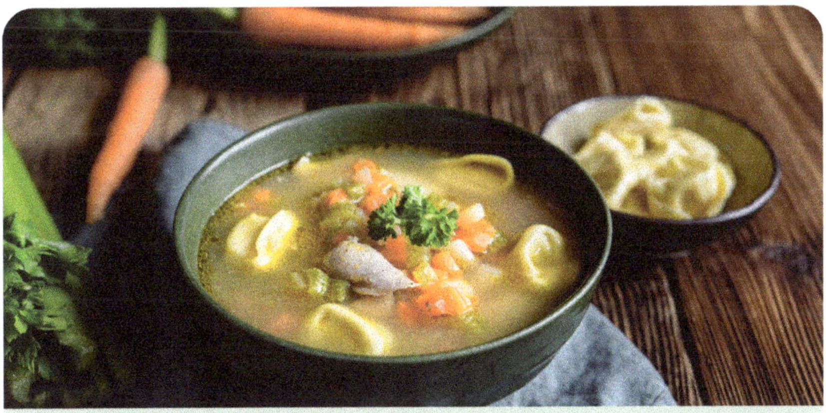

Chicken Tortellini Soup

Serves 4-6

- 1 package organic boneless, skinless chicken thighs (6 thighs)
- Salt or poultry seasoning, to taste
- 1 Tbsp avocado oil or EVOO
- 1 fennel bulb, chopped

- 1 medium onion, chopped
- 2 large carrots, chopped
- 2 parsnips, chopped
- 2-3 cloves garlic, chopped
- 1-2 stalks celery, chopped
- 2 large (32-oz) cartons organic chicken broth
- (1) 15-oz can cannellini or northern beans, drained and rinsed
- 1 package cheese tortellini, uncooked
- 1 bundle of kale or 1 bag of fresh spinach, rinsed and chopped (devein kale if using)
- 2 tbsp fresh parsley
- 1 tsp fresh thyme
- shredded parmesan cheese (optional)
- salt and pepper to taste

Heat the oil in a stock pot. Season the chicken with salt or poultry seasoning, add to the pot, and brown until the center reads 165 degrees on a meat probe. (Or you may grill the chicken if you prefer). Remove the chicken and set aside. Add the chopped garlic, onions, carrots, parsnips, celery, fennel, salt and pepper to the hot oil in the pot (add a bit more oil if needed). Saute until vegetables are tender and onions are translucent. Chop chicken into bite-sized pieces as the veggies are cooking. When they are done, add the broth, chopped chicken, beans, herbs, salt and pepper to the pot. Bring just to a boil and add the tortellini. Cook for about 5 minutes. Add the chopped kale or spinach and cook another 10-15 minutes. To serve, top with a little shredded parmesan cheese if desired. You may make this vegetarian by omitting the chicken and using vegetable broth. Or vegan by further changing the tortellini to a noodle of your choice without the cheese. Enjoy!

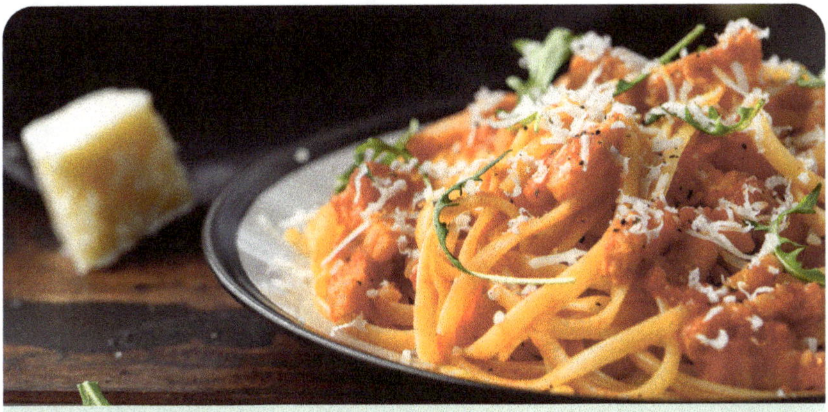

Veggie-Loaded Spaghetti Sauce

Serves 8 or more

- 1 medium onion, chopped
- 1 red bell pepper, copped
- 1 zucchini, chopped
- 1 yellow squash, chopped
- 1 large or 2 smaller carrots, chopped
- 1 smaller eggplant, chopped
- 3 cloves garlic, chopped
- 1 small package baby portabella mushrooms, chopped
- 1 tbsp avocado oil or EVOO
- (2) 15-oz cans tomato sauce
- (1) 28-oz can stewed tomatoes
- fresh or dried basil, parsley and oregano to taste
- 1 bay leaf used during cooking and removed prior to blending
- salt and pepper to taste
- ½ c sweet vermouth (optional secret ingredient)

Heat the oil in a stock pot and add the chopped veggies. Cook until softened and the released water from the veggies is absorbed/evaporated. If using vermouth, add at this time and simmer until liquid is reduced by ½ which will render the alcohol content not a concern in the dish for children. Add the stewed tomatoes, tomato sauce and herbs and simmer for about 30 minutes. Use an emulsion blender to puree the chunks into a smooth sauce right in the pot. Serve over the pasta of your choice.

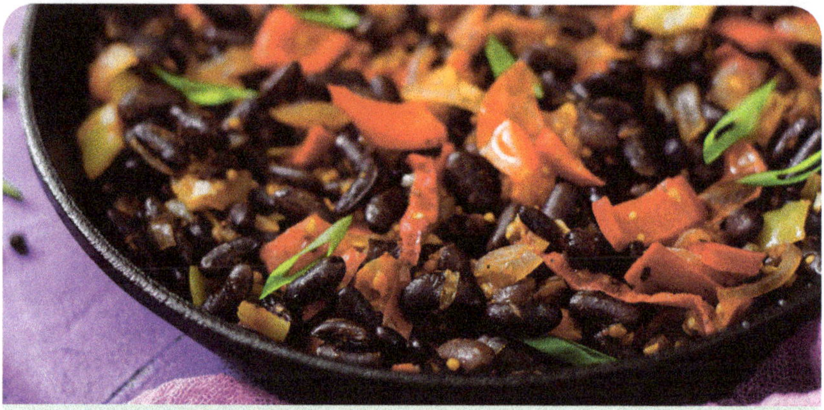

Chunky Veggie and Bean Chili

Serves 6-8

- 1 medium onion, chopped
- 1 red bell pepper, chopped
- 3 cloves garlic, chopped
- 1 zucchini, chopped
- 1 yellow squash, chopped
- 1 large carrot, chopped
- 1 baby eggplant, chopped
- (1) 15-oz can tomato sauce
- (1) 15-oz can diced tomatoes

- (1) 15-oz can vegetable broth
- 1 tbsp avocado oil or EVOO
- (1) 15-oz can each dark-red kidney beans, light-red kidney beans, and black beans, drained and rinsed
- 2 tbsp chili powder, 1 tbsp cumin, 1 tsp salt and ½ tsp black pepper.
- 1 chipotle chili in adobo sauce or other chilis of your choice (optional, if you like more spice)

Heat the oil in a stock pot and add the chopped veggies. Cook over med-med high heat until softened and the released water is absorbed/evaporated, stir often to avoid browning the veggies and ensure even cooking. This will take approximately 25-30 minutes (because there's a lot of veggies!) . Add spices and mix to release the aromatics for 1 minute then add remaining ingredients. Bring to a gentle boil then cover and reduce to simmer for about 30 minutes or more to allow the flavors to meld. You can also add cooked drained lean ground meat or lentils for a meaty texture if desired. If adding lentils either precook according to package instructions or add ½ c rinsed brown lentils with the beans and an additional 1c water or broth. Serve with whole grain rolls.

Using cooked rutabaga for half or all of the potatoes in potato salad is an easy way to decrease carbohydrates and introduce a wider range of minerals, vitamins and antioxidants. Spiral-cut zucchini and summer squash are perfect as a noodle replacement in raw form, using your traditional sauces on top. These are quick and easy to prepare with markedly fewer calories and, again, more variety. Pulse-blend raw cauliflower to produce a unique substitute for rice in Asian dishes (or mix half and half with your rice). Use raw avocado or hummus as a spread on your usual turkey sandwich or roll-up. This can be in addition to what you already do - it doesn't have to be a substitute. Think variety: An "add in" can be as good as a replacement in many situations, and the more plant-based products added, the better.

Add more variety to your salads, too. Try fruits such as oranges, strawberries, pears or pomegranate seeds. Nuts such as almonds, walnuts and pine nuts are a great complement to greens, as are sunflower seeds, which are high in protein, vitamin E and fiber. Buy your lettuce whole, and make your own greens mixes to save money over the prepackaged kinds. Mix raw spinach and romaine or leaf lettuce and even consider adding raw herbs like fresh parsley, dill or basil if you like for a twist. Raw kale is wonderful for salads, but it is always better if you "massage" it before using - really. After thoroughly washing and trimming out the center spine, put a little oil in your palm with some coarse salt and crush the kale between your hands until soft and bright green. Then chop it into small pieces and top with your choice of goodies - nuts and dried berries go very well here. Adding garbanzo beans and some cooked whole grains like quinoa, barley or wheat berries (which is the entire wheat kernel including the endosperm, germ and bran) adds a wonderfully hearty quality.

You can also "healthify" recipes by making substitutions for less healthy ingredients. This is easiest in baked goods - for example, using applesauce in place of vegetable oil and/or low-fat plain yogurt in place of sour cream, both in equal measurements. Try using two egg whites in place of one whole egg. I often use "chia eggs" in baked goods or even if using a store-bought muffin mix. You may be able to find commercial versions of these mixes that use natural ingredients, but it is easy and less expensive to make your own. For a chia egg, simply mix one tablespoon of chia seeds with three tablespoons of water and leave to soak for about 10 minutes. Stir periodically, and the mixture will turn gelatinous and can serve as a substitute for one egg. This is yet another way to incorporate a wider variety of nutrients. Chia seeds (often referred to as a superfood) are very high in fiber, omega-3 fatty acids, protein, antioxidants, vitamins and minerals. They are crunchy when dry and can be a great addition to homemade granola or cereal, and gelatinous when mixed with liquid. I also commonly make chia pudding, which is similar in consistency to tapioca. You can make it with the milk of your choice, raw honey or pure maple syrup, and pure vanilla, cinnamon or even pure cocoa. There are endless recipes online with suggestions for using chia seeds. However, do NOT consume a large amount (spoonful) of plain raw DRY chia seeds as they can expand in the esophagus and lead to choking. Believe it or not, another "healthification" you can do is to use pureed black beans in place of flour in brownie recipes - really, no one will be able to tell the difference!

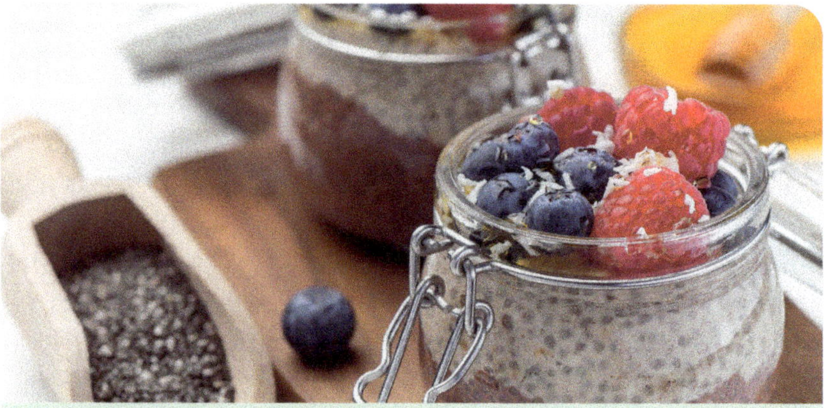

Vanilla Chia Pudding

Serves 3-4

- 1 ¾ c almond, soy or coconut milk
- 2 tsp vanilla extract
- ⅓ c chia seeds
- 3 tbsp maple syrup or honey
- Berries for topping (optional)

Place all ingredients in a Mason jar, screw the lid on tightly, and shake to mix very well (or stir well in a bowl and cover). Refrigerate for 60 minutes or more until thickened, stir well after approximately 15 minutes, 30 minutes and again prior to serving. Top with berries if desired.

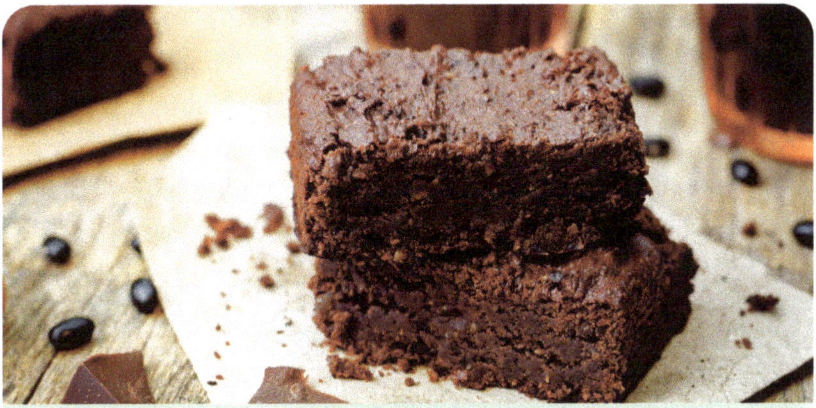

Black Bean Brownies

Makes 9 thin brownies

- (1) 15-oz can of black beans, drained and rinsed
- 3 eggs or egg substitute
- 3 tbsp avocado oil
- 1 tsp vanilla
- ¼ c unsweetened cocoa powder
- ⅔ c sugar
- ½ tsp baking powder
- ¼ tsp salt
- ½ c chocolate chips (optional)

Preheat oven to 350 degrees. Grease an 8" x 8" pan or line with parchment paper. Puree black beans in a food processor into a rough paste. Mix the puree with the eggs, oil and vanilla in a large bowl. In a separate bowl, mix the cocoa powder, sugar, baking powder and salt and add to the wet ingredients. Stir in chocolate chips if using. Pour mixture into prepared pan and bake for 30-40 minutes until the edges are visibly cooked and a toothpick inserted into the center comes out clean. Allow to cool prior to cutting.

Black beans are also delicious in vegetarian burgers, as a dip, or in hummus as mentioned earlier. It doesn't have to be all or nothing, either. You can start by doing a half substitution. For example, instead of replacing all the oil in the muffin recipe with applesauce, do half and half - or even less. Ease your way into it. Especially when altering sauces, starting with small additions will be less noticeable to kids, and then as the exposure adjusts their palate, you can add more and more. The same applies to decreasing sugar in recipes - start slowly and gradually cut back more. If you are not successful in the beginning, don't let that discourage you. It's like running: You can't run a marathon on day one, and you likely won't win them all. But that's OK.

Many people are unaware of the numerous health benefits of hulled hemp seed hearts. Yes, they come from the cannabis plant, but they do not contain THC (the main psychoactive compound in cannabis). They are technically a nut, and have a mild nutty flavor. They contain two essential fatty acids, omega-3 and omega-6, and 25 percent of their total calories are from high-quality protein. They are also a great source of vitamin E and minerals and can be used raw, cooked or roasted. Adding these to your baked goods or raw snacks is a great way to "healthify." Interestingly, hemp seed oil has been used as a medicine in China for at least 3000 years, so it certainly isn't something new. It's just coming back full circle.

I have to admit that I have made rice crispy treats and have added hemp seed hearts raw, without anyone noticing. I usually use them for power protein balls or raw or baked cookies or muffins. The power protein balls are great on-the-go snacks for kids, especially prior to sports or exercise.

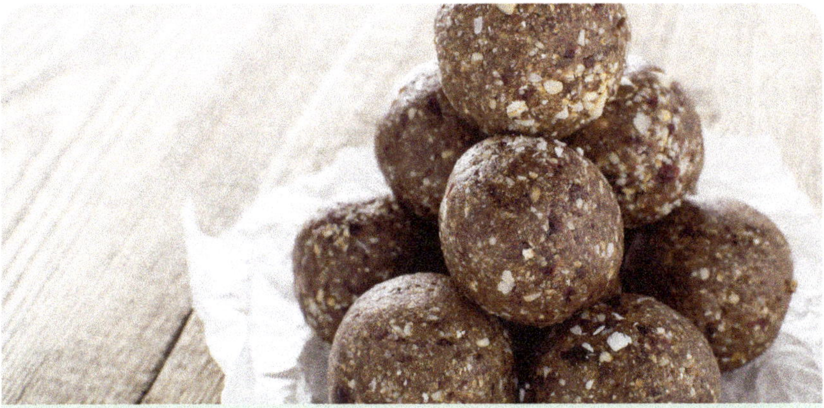

No-Bake Power Protein Balls

Servings vary

- ¾ c old-fashioned rolled oats
- ½ c almond flour
- 1 tbsp cinnamon
- 1 tbsp chia seeds
- 1 tbsp hulled hemp seeds (available in health food stores or large grocery chains)
- 1 tbsp flax seeds
- ¼ c peanut butter (or other nut butter)
- ¼ c raw honey
- 1 tsp vanilla
- 1 tbsp unrefined coconut oil (melted)

Mix oats, almond flour, cinnamon, chia seeds, hulled hemp seeds and flax seeds in a blender or food processor and process to a flour like consistency. Transfer to a large bowl. Combine the nut butter, raw honey, vanilla extract and coconut oil in another bowl and add to the dry ingredients. Mix together well. (This takes a little time, so be patient.) Roll the mixture into small balls about 1-inch in diameter, arrange them on a parchment-lined cookie sheet, and place in the freezer for 30 minutes (more is ok) so they won't stick together. Remove them from the cookie sheet and store them in a lidded plastic container in the refrigerator. (They will be good for at least a few weeks, but they never last that long in our house!) You can use maple syrup instead of honey and add cocoa if you like - there are many options here for variety.

Silken tofu is a great product to use for pudding. I know it may sound odd, and I am actually not much of a fan of cooked tofu or tempeh (kudos to those of you who are), however there are some recipes where it really is ideal in this completely different form.

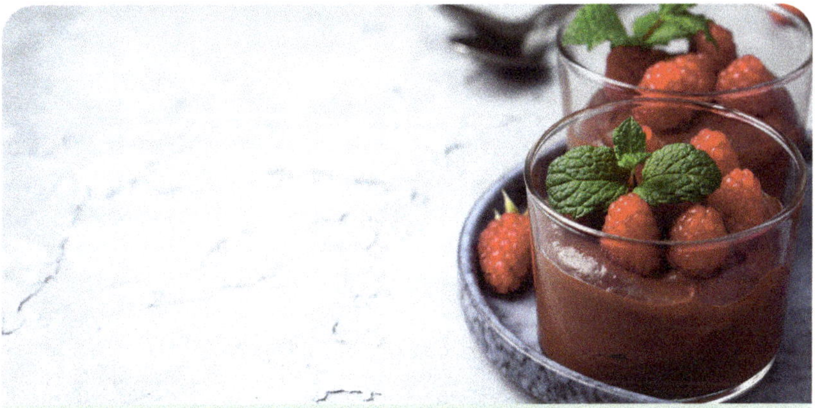

Plant Based Chocolate Pudding

Makes 3-4 small servings

- 1½ cups raw silken tofu
- ⅓ cup pure cocoa
- ⅓ cup pure maple syrup
- 2 teaspoons vanilla

Simply add all ingredients to a food processor and blend until smooth. Chill in the refrigerator for 30 min or until ready to serve. I usually add a few fresh raspberries on top when serving. I have received rave reviews on this dessert from people who would never have tried it if they had known it had tofu in it! Silken tofu is great in smoothies too, which brings us to our next chapter.

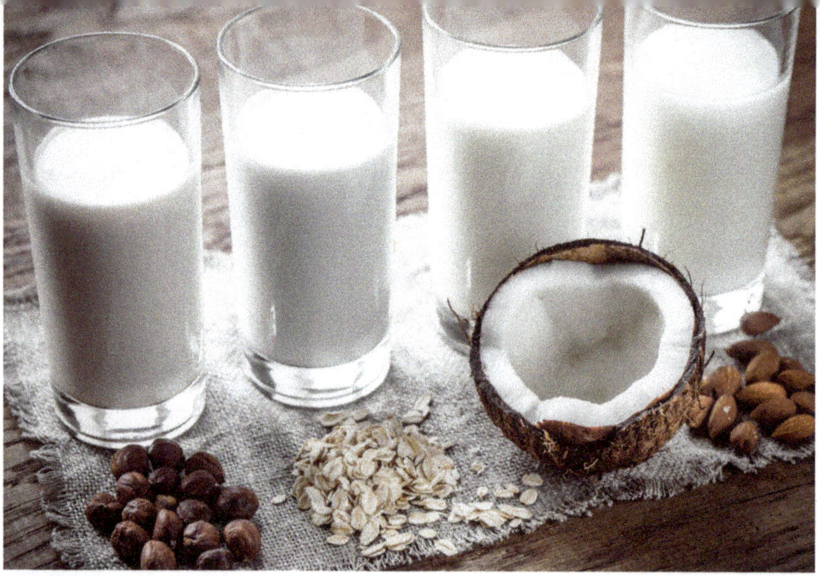

HOW:

MILKS/SMOOTHIES

Using a variety of milks is another easy way to introduce a variety of different proteins, fats, antioxidants, vitamins and minerals into your family's diet. Note that it is important to avoid added sugar when you are purchasing any kind of milk, including plant-based. If you choose to use cow's milk, try to use organic. The belief that children must have cow's milk every day to be healthy is a farce propagated by the dairy industry through a very successful marketing campaign. Kids do need healthy proteins and fats, but these do not have to come from a cow. Humans have no nutritional requirement for animal milk, an evolutionary recent addition to our diet. Many populations throughout the world today consume little or no milk for biological reasons (lactose intolerance or allergy), lack of availability, or cultural preferences. Adequate dietary calcium for bone health, often cited as the primary rationale for high intake of milk, can be obtained from other sources. A document published in 2014 reviewed over 400 reputable scientific papers concluded that not only is animal milk not necessary, but in many ways it is harmful.[25, 56] Frank Oski, former pediatric surgery director at Johns Hopkins School of Medicine reported that one-half of all iron deficiency in infants in the U.S. is due to milk-induced gastrointestinal bleeding (often microscopic and not visible) due to an allergy to the protein casein.[26]

Most pasteurized milk sold at supermarkets comes from concentrated animal feeding operations (CAFOs), where the animals may be fed antibiotics. They may also receive hormones, in an effort to increase milk production, and they are fed a diet of grains and soy rather than grass, which alters their gut flora (good bacteria) and the nutritional quality of the milk. Choosing organic dairy (milk, sour cream, cheese, butter, etc.) will help to avoid these antibiotic and hormone containing cow's milk products. I'll bet you are thinking, "Can't I just go to the store and buy food without all this confusion?" Not anymore, unfortunately. Our country has become dominated by big business and government lobbying, and our quality of food, safety and health has suffered as a consequence. If you have access to a local farm where you can purchase your meat and dairy, know their practices and can confirm the quality of their products, that is certainly the best way to go. Support your local farmers!

Some people consume *raw* animal milk and tout its health benefits. While it is true that many micronutrients are destroyed either partially or completely through the heating process of pasteurization, this has also been a necessary measure due to serious risks associated with bacterial contamination of milk. Certainly any potential benefits of raw animal milk would not outweigh the risks.

A2 milk is a form of cow's milk that is reported to be better tolerated in those who report an intolerance to lactose. A portion of the protein in cow's milk is known as beta-casein. Historically, all beta-casein was in the form of A2. Currently it is in the form of A1 and A2. The A2 protein is more similar to that found in human breast milk, as well as goat, sheep and buffalo milks. Certain studies have reported fewer incidences of gastrointestinal symptoms in those who consume the A2 milk. It is thought that in these people, it may not be lactose as the underlying source of their intolerance, but rather the A1 protein.[26]

Fortunately for those who choose to avoid all animal milks, there are currently many other options available, including almond, cashew, soy, rice, coconut, hemp, oat, flaxseed and even peanut milk. We certainly know water is the best beverage for everyone, but there are health benefits to consider that can be obtained from plant beverages as well. And even if your child doesn't like almond milk in cold cereal, for example, you could still use it to make cooked oatmeal or smoothies. Try to use an assortment of different plant-based milks for more variety, rather than sticking to only one kind. Different milks contain an array of different proteins, fats and other nutrients, so dabble in them all unless you or any members of your family are restricted due to allergies.

One downfall of store-bought plant milks, however, is that they tend to have additives and emulsifiers, are often quite dilute and thus less nutritious, use blanched nuts, and/or are pasteurized, which destroys many beneficial antioxidants, as mentioned earlier. Therefore, I recommend making your own plant milk! It is so easy and so much more nutritious. You can save money, too, when you get your ingredients from the bulk foods section of your grocery store.

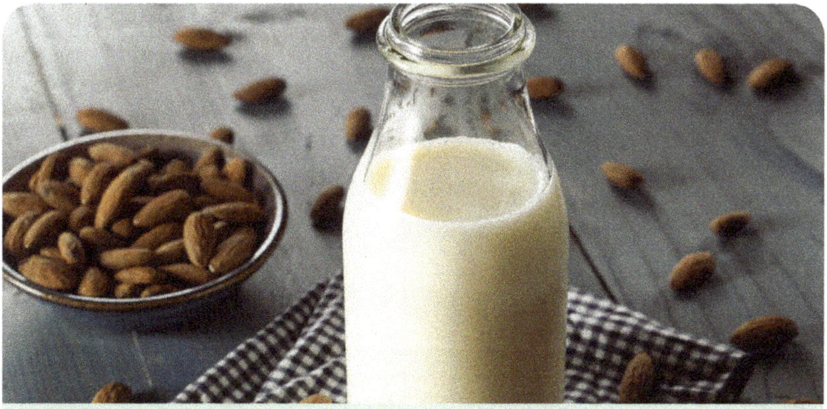

Almond Milk

Makes 1 quart

- I c raw (unblanched) almonds
- 4 c fresh filtered water, plus more for soaking
- 1-2 pitted dates (optional)
- 1 tsp vanilla (optional)

Despite the almonds' brown skins, your milk will be perfectly white. Cover the nuts with water in a bowl or a Mason jar and soak for several hours or overnight. (Cashews and oats do not need to soak, but do rinse them). Drain the water and put the nuts in a good-quality blender. Add the fresh filtered water and blend for two minutes. You may add a pitted date or two as a natural sweetener or add a teaspoon of pure vanilla for flavor if you like. Strain the pureed liquid through cheesecloth or a nut-milk bag (readily available online or from many health food stores). Store the milk in the refrigerator for a maximum of 5 to 6 days. It will naturally separate, so just shake before serving. It's that easy!

In our family, we often use our homemade almond milk for overnight oatmeal. Each family member can make his or her own version, too. Letting the whole raw oats soak overnight allows them to develop a creamy texture, as if they were slow-cooked. They can be eaten raw in the morning or heated in the microwave. It's a fast and easy breakfast and unique to each individual.

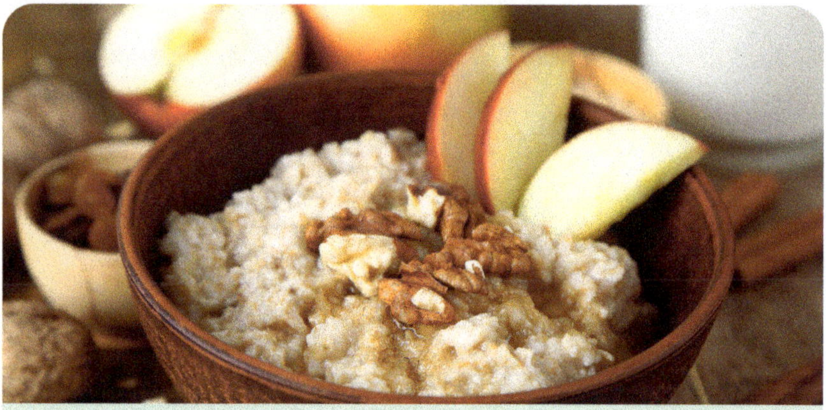

Cinnamon-Apple Overnight Oatmeal Recipe

Serves 1

- 1 c old fashioned rolled oats
- 1 c milk of choice (more or less as desired)
- 1 tsp chia seeds (available at health food stores or large grocery chains)
- 1 tsp raw honey or maple syrup
- ¼ c finely chopped raw apple
- ½ tsp cinnamon

Mix all ingredients, pour into a container that will easily hold all of the ingredients, cover, and refrigerate overnight. If a hot oatmeal is desired simply heat in the microwave for 1 ½ minutes and stir well. You could also add raisins, dried cranberries or nuts. Other varieties could include berries, bananas, pureed pumpkin, yougurt or applesauce. Using chopped pitted dates or vanilla can also add more variety.

Smoothies are another great way to add variety to kids' diets. I have introduced these as early as eight to nine months of age. The sky's the limit with options. Usually, starting with a ripe banana is helpful, as it lends natural sweetness to the drink. From there, you could add frozen or fresh strawberries, raspberries, cranberries, blueberries, blackberries, cherries, acai berries (frozen puree-unsweetened) and/or other fruits of preference. Generally, adding a yogurt and or milk of your choice gives a pleasant texture to the drink. Some people prefer to use ice and tropical fruits such as mango, pineapple or papaya. Pure coconut water or aloe juice are other liquids that may be used. There are no limits, but I do recommend avoiding added sugar. If the drink is a bit tart, consider adding some pure raw honey instead.

If after making a smoothie, you find you have extra, freezing it into a popsicle mold is a great way to save it. Even if kids are not fond of a particular smoothie, they will often accept it in popsicle form. Smoothies are a great way to introduce various kinds of produce into your children's diet. Spinach is often very well tolerated, as is avocado, with its very smooth texture and a mild taste, and silken tofu, as mentioned earlier. But sometimes you may need to come up with creative discussions regarding the color of a smoothie in order for your child to accept it. For example, I have heard parents say they use a different color smoothie for each day of the week. (Or you can put it in a dark cup with a lid)

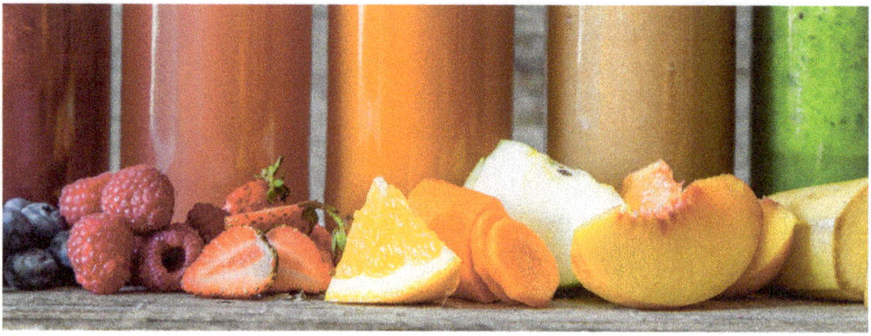

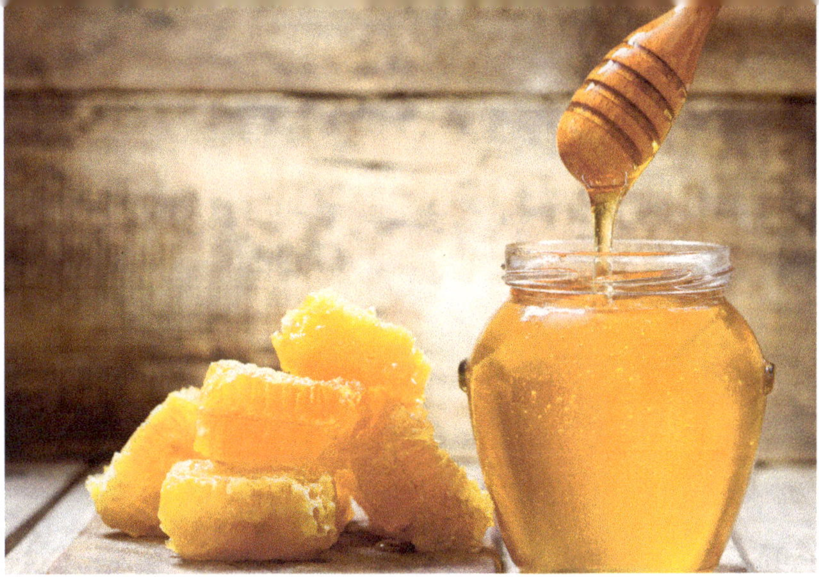

HOW:

SWEETENERS

Varying sweeteners is another good thing to implement in gradually making healthy adjustments to your family's diet. Avoiding refined white sugar and high fructose corn syrup (HFCS) is certainly recommended due to increased rates of obesity, diabetes, heart disease and cancer in those consuming these in high amounts. Many everyday foods and beverages contain one or both of these ingredients. Obvious culprits are soda/pop and candy, but sugar and/or HFCS is commonly found in processed foods like sweetened yogurts, many salad dressings, frozen TV dinners/pizzas and snack foods, many bread products, canned fruit (choose fruit in its natural juices) and some frozen and dried fruits as well, juice drinks, boxed meal kits with powdered sauces and seasonings, granola bars, breakfast cereals, store-bought baked goods, store-bought BBQ sauce and ketchup, many condiments, chips, snack bars, artificially flavored fruit snacks, cookies, donuts, chocolate milk and cocoa...and the list goes on.

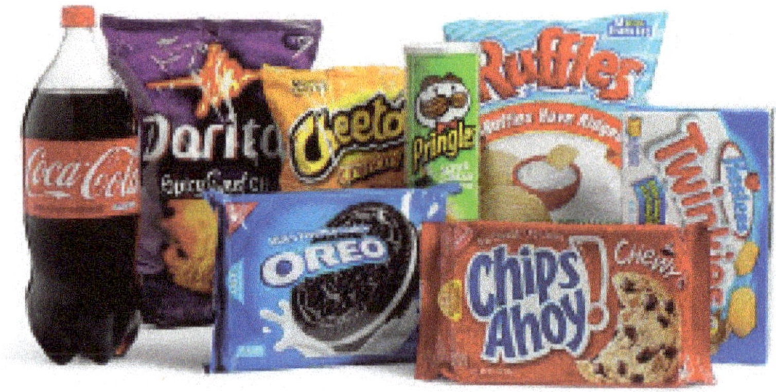

Certain natural sweeteners have some health benefits when they have not been highly processed. Raw honey has many antioxidants, antibacterial and antifungal properties and has been used to heal wounds in Europe. There are reports of it being effective against bacteria such as MRSA (resistant Staphylococcus aureus causing several kinds of infections) and Helicobacter pylori (a common cause of gastrointestinal ulcers, which in some cases untreated can increase the risk for gastric or stomach cancer). Note however, that you must not give any honey to babies under one year of age due to the risk of botulism - a serious infectious disease, also termed *floppy baby syndrome*.

Pure maple syrup also has many antioxidants as well as vitamins and minerals, including zinc and manganese, which are important for a healthy immune system. This does not include syrups made from corn syrup or refined processed honey. It is worth saving money on expensive vitamins and supplements (as these are typically highly processed as well) and rather spending it on much higher quality natural foods. For adults following a whole food diet, this often results in fewer medication costs, as mentioned earlier.

Having the whole family on the same page regarding meals and nutrition is very important, since children follow our lead. Keep in mind however, that for those with diabetes, *all* sweeteners need to be limited, as the body treats them similarly with regard to blood glucose levels. Also, while there may be some benefits to using raw honey, pure maple syrup or coconut sugar instead of refined granulated sugar, an excess of any of these is best avoided. And artificial "zero-calorie" sweeteners are not a good substitute. We will discuss this further in the next chapter on beverages. The fact is that the more sugary foods we consume, the more we crave them. It is clear that whether the sweetened item is real sugar or a zero-calorie sweetener, the individual continues to crave more sweet products, vs. those who avoid sweet items altogether.

In summary, there are many potential issues here regarding sweeteners:

- Empty calories with no nutritional value with simple processed sugar
- Better nutritional value overall with natural sugars such as raw honey, pure maple syrup and dates, but still excess calories, risks for diabetics and weight gain, as well as tooth decay (all seen with simple sugar, too)
- Artificial sweeteners - increased weight gain despite being calorie-free, due to increased sweet cravings and other factors, as well as some concerns of increased carcinogenicity effects

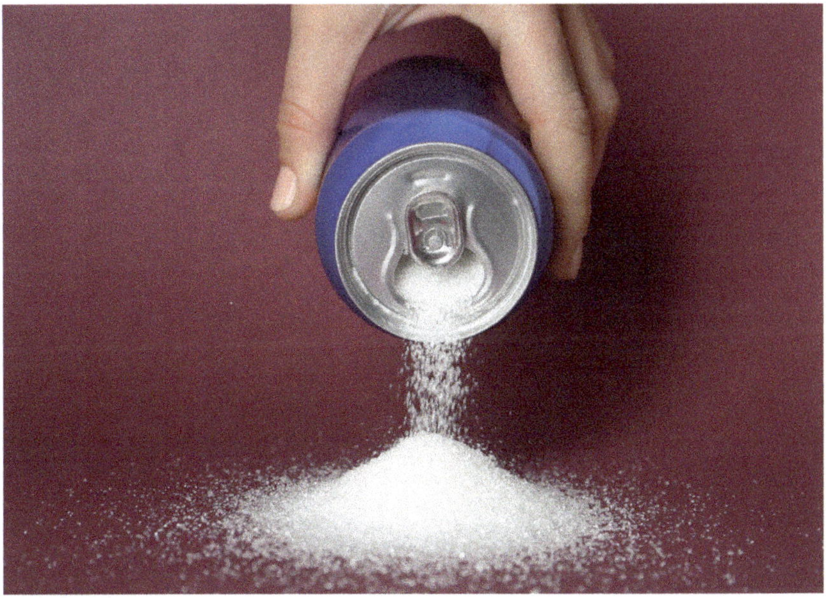

HOW:

BEVERAGES

Children consume alarming amounts of sugar in beverages. This leads to dental disease, inappropriate weight gain, mood changes and an increased risk of diabetes. Frequent use of sugary foods is clearly associated with decreased acceptance of healthy fresh foods. Sodas are harmful in more ways than sugar - for example, some contain caffeine, which is not appropriate for children. Carbonation contains an acidic solution which in excessive amounts can cause heartburn, gastric (stomach) ulcers, dental disease, abdominal bloating (gas), and decreased bone density. As mentioned previously, diet beverages are not a good replacement. Most contain artificial sweeteners, and even if it is one that is natural, it has a much higher potency of sweetness than regular sugar. Therefore, although we are not gaining calories from this, we are developing a heightened tolerance to sweetness and thus crave more sweets, contributing to a vicious cycle that has been linked with higher rates of diabetes and metabolic syndrome compared to those who consume water.

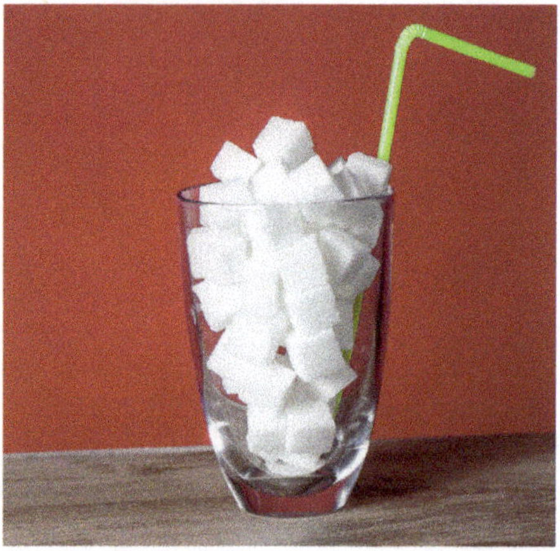

Oftentimes, well-meaning parents allow their children to drink chocolate milk, pleased with the low fat labeling (this pertains to cow *and* plant based milks). But they are often unaware that just 4 ounces (½ cup) contain 25 grams of sugar - that's more than 6 teaspoons in that little box on their child's lunch tray! Thankfully, more and more schools are removing this option in the best interest of our children. Encouraging them to drink a glass of water prior to drinking any other beverage is helpful in reducing the consumption of sugary beverages. Stand firm, because you will see that after drinking that glass of water, your child will usually no longer be thirsty and will have forgotten about the other drink and have moved on. Sometimes we need to use some psychology on those little ones!

Especially with older adolescents, infusing water can make it more attractive/palatable. Placing some cut-up, peeled cucumbers or a handful of blueberries or fresh mint in a pitcher of cold water in the fridge can add a unique twist that may be more acceptable to them. Flavored carbonated waters without sweeteners of any kind are better than soda, certainly, but you do want to watch the quantities of these as well. The pluses are that they are without caffeine, sodium, sugar, artificial sweeteners and artificial flavors. But due to the carbonation, they are acidic in pH, which is damaging to the teeth as well as the stomach lining. So again, try to keep those beverages infrequent - and if you do offer them, consider decreasing the quantity by sharing a can or bottle amongst the kids, and try to have them brush their teeth soon after consuming it.

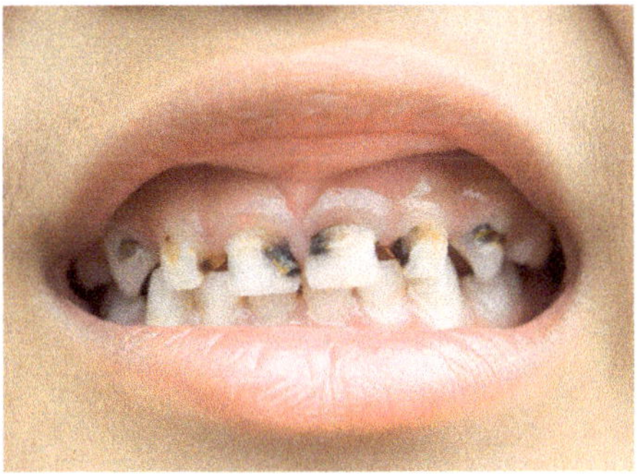

If you do choose to use a "sweet" beverage, try to avoid anything other than 100 percent juice. Be aware, though, that even shopping for something as simple as juice can be very misleading. Pay attention to labels - they may include phrases like "all natural" or "no additives or preservatives" or "contains real juice." These statements do not equate to a statement of 100 percent juice. You may see "juice drink," too, and this is not real juice. These products often contain artificial colors and flavors as well. You will also see labels touting "less sugar." This is impossible - you cannot remove natural sugar from 100 percent juice. These are cases in which manufacturers take 100 percent juice, dilute it with water by up to 50 percent, and sell it to you at the same price as the undiluted version. Or worse, they will dilute it and add artificial sweeteners. So if you choose to drink that kind of juice, buy the real stuff and dilute it yourself. Even with that, try to use a fruit/vegetable blend, a low-sodium vegetable juice (it doesn't have to be tomato, e.g., it can be carrot or another kind), or try pure coconut water. In any case, limit all of these drinks to no more than 4-8 ounces per day. Or better yet, try juicing yourself!

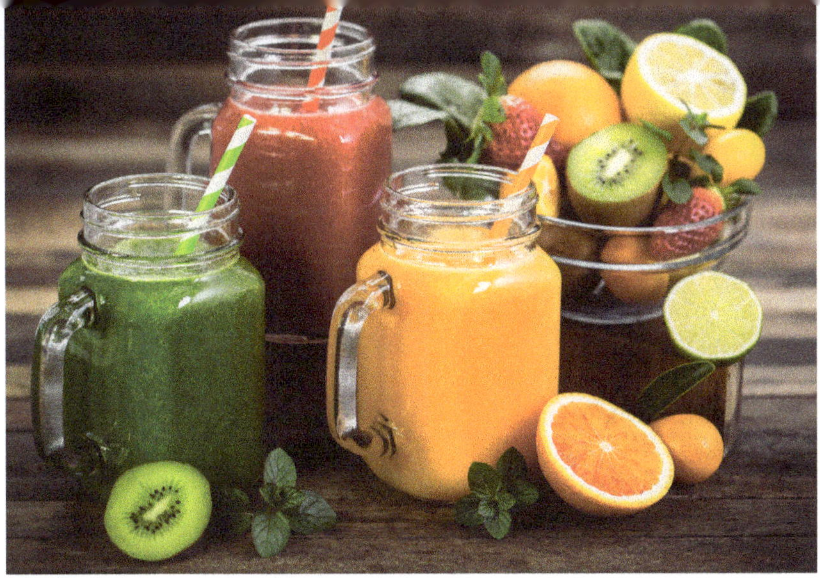

HOW:

JUICING

Juicing has great health benefits, but also some potential negatives to be aware of. Generally speaking, juicing fresh fruits - and especially vegetables - is a very healthy choice for most children and adults. It is a great way to concentrate many vitamins, minerals, antioxidants and other nutrients in their most natural, unaltered form. When prepared fresh and consumed immediately, these juices are not subject to destructive elements such as water, light and heat, which are the norm for commercially produced juices. This is a wonderful way to introduce and obtain the health benefits of foods that might otherwise be absent from your child's diet.

Of course, if your child loves grapes, plums, carrots and beans, by all means, have him or her eat them in whole form. And use juicing to incorporate fruits or vegetables that are *less* preferred, mixed with some that your child likes a lot. I often juice oranges, lemon, lime, sweet potato, carrot, zucchini, summer squash and apple or pear - all together. The citrus packs a punch and the apple/pear adds natural sweetness. Adding greens is great, and spinach in particular is well tolerated. Some people like to include the peel (or part of the peel) of citrus fruits, but that can be overpowering for children. Certain foods can dominate the flavor of the juice, which may or may not be desired. Examples of this would be beets, celery, herbs such as parsley, and roots like ginger. There are endless recipes you can use, depending on your family's palates, and you can use more of certain flavors and less of others to gradually introduce variety.

One important principle here is to use organic foods whenever possible, or peel your produce if it is not organic. You do not want to concentrate pesticides by juicing. Another factor to consider is that the fiber is removed from the foods through juicing, therefore it will not sustain fullness. This is *not* a good choice for those intending to lose weight, or those with diabetes. However, from the point of view of trying to maximize nutrient consumption in a plant-based form, juicing is a great way to do this. It is not intended as a replacement for consuming whole fruits and vegetables, but rather more as a "supplement," or a way to consume additional vitamins and minerals and other micronutrients from a variety of fresh produce *above and beyond* what you are able to consume in whole form. You can also compost the pulp from juicing for your garden. The juice is not intended to be saved for later, so make only what you plan to consume immediately. It can be expensive and requires time for preparation and cleaning, but it is still so worth it in my opinion.

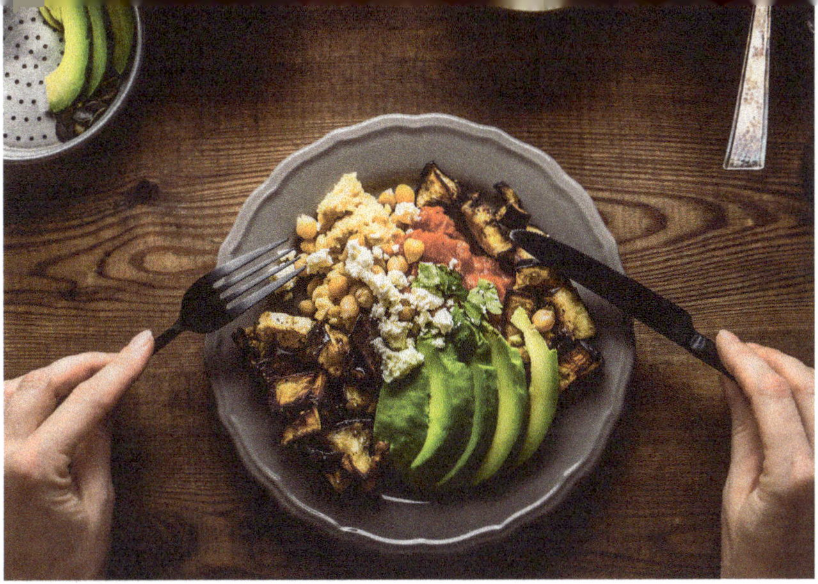

HOW:

EATING OUT

There are always times when we need to, or want to eat out. Be aware that when eating out menus often include foods that contain very high amounts of hidden fats, sugar, sodium and in some/many cases the artificial colors, flavors, preservatives and pesticides that we referred to earlier. In small, infrequent quantities these substances are likely of no significant health concern, however cumulatively, in larger quantities, they present a potentially substantial risk to our health. Choosing local reputable restaurants is key, because they are more likely to provide clean food options. What I mean by "clean" is food that is more likely freshly made with higher-quality ingredients. Many chain restaurants premake their products and ship them packaged or frozen. They are more likely to use meat from CAFOs (confined animal feeding operations) and farmed fish, both of which we will talk about in the chapter *WHAT ABOUT: MEAT AND FISH.* They are also more likely to use produce that has been shipped across the country, increasing handling and food contamination risks. And they tend to use the lower-quality processed oils we discussed earlier. They commonly use syrup made from high-fructose corn syrup with artificial flavors, colors and preservatives. They also frequently serve juice drinks instead of real juice, and grains are commonly highly processed - not whole grain. All of these factors can easily go unrecognized when placing an order for a meal. Therefore, it not only matters *what* you eat, but also *where* you eat.

When eating out with children, it can be helpful to bring some fresh fruits or raw vegetables from home to add to their meal. Often, there may be an option for a side dish. Have each child choose a different side - such as broccoli and grapes - and split it with his or her sibling, adding variety. The same could apply to the main dish, with maybe a meat and a red sauce pasta, for example. Split it and have less meat for each child and more variety. As adults, you might also want to consider sharing sides for variety.

Many restaurants have very poor choices on children's menus. Because of this, you might want to consider ordering a dish or an appetizer from the adult menu that is a healthier choice for the kids to split. For example, a hummus appetizer, a baked fish dish, certain soups and salads, veggie potstickers or edamame (soybeans). Salad bars are generally good options, too, since everyone can pick and choose which items they like. The kids might prefer plain tomatoes, cucumbers, cottage cheese or other familiar items. It can be quite challenging eating out with children, hence its better and cheaper to cook at home! The good news is, so far I have not seen problems with restaurants up charging when meal-splitting for kids.

One thing my kids have enjoyed from eating out and that we have implemented at home is "courses." I generally give them fruit for what we call their first course. It may be grapes, apples, mango, berries, kiwi, watermelon, peaches or a combination of fruits. Their second course is always a vegetable - usually a salad or chopped-up raw veggies and a balsamic drizzle. Their third course is the main entree. Occasionally, we will do a fourth course of a dessert, which I usually try to make a healthy treat. They find this fun, and I find it convenient, since I can still be preparing the main course while they have started their fruit. As we all know, kids tend to be slow eaters, and this helps so that their hot food doesn't get cold while they are poking at their salad. Although with that, there is of course a delay in the whole family eating together. Do as you see fit. I find that having the children and their parents in close proximity and cooking/eating/discussing food is adequate for the first part of dinner. Then we join together for the main course. Skip desserts - keep them a rare treat. Eat slowly, as we tend to eat too much when we eat too fast. Drink water first, socialize and take your time. Digestion does not like to be rushed. And the heart and soul needs to slow down and enjoy the company too.

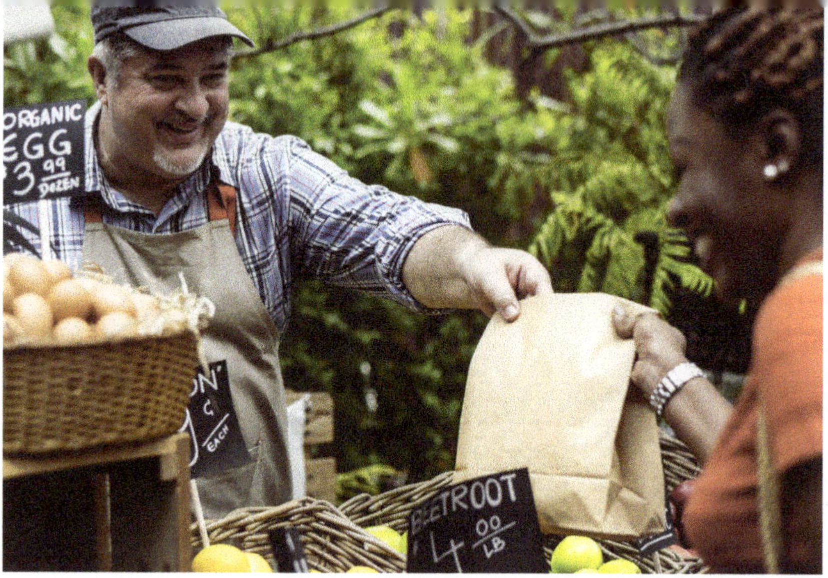

HOW:

FRESH PRODUCE

Fresh is always best, but not always necessary. For example, we know fresh beans and peas have a very short life span once picked and therefore are commonly fresh-frozen. This is the case with fresh berries as well. Frozen or even canned produce is better than none, but fresh, *and local,* is best. The reason for this is that produce from other states or countries is picked early to ripen during transit. We know that food allowed to ripen on the vine is much more nutrient rich as well as more flavorful. Hence the desire to obtain locally grown produce. The cost is also more affordable when produce is purchased in season. That's why having your asparagus in the spring is cheap and plentiful and squashes are best in the fall/winter. Paying attention to seasonal availability of produce is key - this has been the way our ancestors fed themselves for centuries. Pay attention to recommendations on how best to store your produce as well (e.g. tomatoes, bananas and avocados should not be refrigerated). Using seasonal availability of produce as a guide to your home meal menu is very helpful.

Many people choose to join a CSA (Community Sponsored Agriculture) when shopping for farm-fresh food. This is a

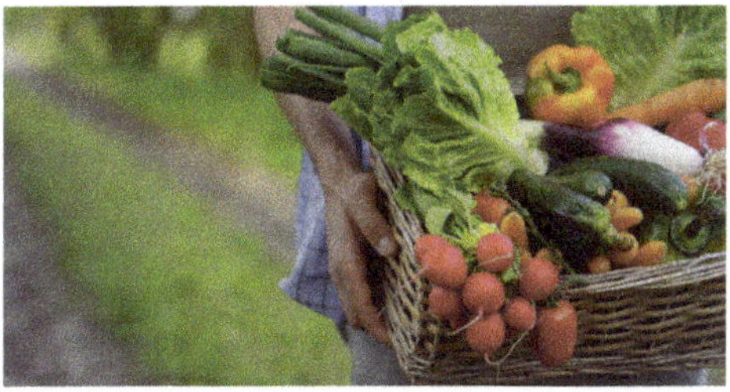

wonderful way to enjoy a variety of abundant local produce. For a set fee, local farmers will provide a share of their crop weekly during the season, and depending on the productivity of the year, some shares may be much more plentiful than others. You consume local fresh produce throughout the growing season while supporting your local farmers. For our family, it has been a great way for us to learn new ways to use produce or try new things. For example, we had a year when there was an abundance of radishes. Now while I love raw radishes, there are only so many one can consume in a sitting. Therefore my husband, a die-hard griller at heart, decided to grill them for us. Low and behold, they were wonderful and lost all their spiciness (which was a good thing for this batch). Had we not received the large quantity of radishes that week in our CSA, we wouldn't have reached beyond our boundaries to explore something new. And the list of benefits go on with a CSA. I am a strong supporter.

Outside our growing season, fortunately for those of us in the north, it is a blessing that we have produce available year-round from imports despite our cold winter climate. Otherwise, in the winter we would mostly rely on canned and pickled produce, which can be a concern for those following low-sodium (reduced-salt) diets. The reason fresh is best is that with time after picking, light, water and heat leach or destroy many of the vitamins, minerals and antioxidants naturally found in produce. This is also why, generally speaking, raw is better than broiling/grilling, which is better than steaming, which is better than boiling/stewing (including crock pots). Similarly, it is best to avoid pre-washed, chopped and prepared "convenience" foods, as they tend to cost more and have a shorter shelf life - not very convenient! Those products often carry a higher risk of food poisoning as well, due to handling and the false perception that they do not need to be washed. Never trust that. Always wash your produce right when you need to use it.

If you live in an area that allows you to grow your own garden, do whatever you can to make that happen. If you start your garden from seed, it is very inexpensive. But even if you don't, having your own garden is economical and very rewarding. Certainly it requires a lot of work, but most people who grow gardens find that they obtain more physical activity (which most of us need more of), and they find contentment and relaxation in their work.

Vegetable gardens can and often do include flowers as well, which serve not only as a decorative feature, but some act as a natural insect repellent. Going out to your garden to pick fresh food to use for your meal is very fulfilling. One idea that some parents might want to adopt would be planting a "pizza garden." This may include things one could put on a pizza, such as tomatoes, onions, bell peppers, spinach, basil, oregano, or any other desired ingredients. If your residence cannot accommodate a garden, there are often community gardens that you may be able to participate in. Involvement in growing food is very beneficial for children. They not only learn this important skill, but also learn to appreciate freshly harvested food over processed food, which is so important.

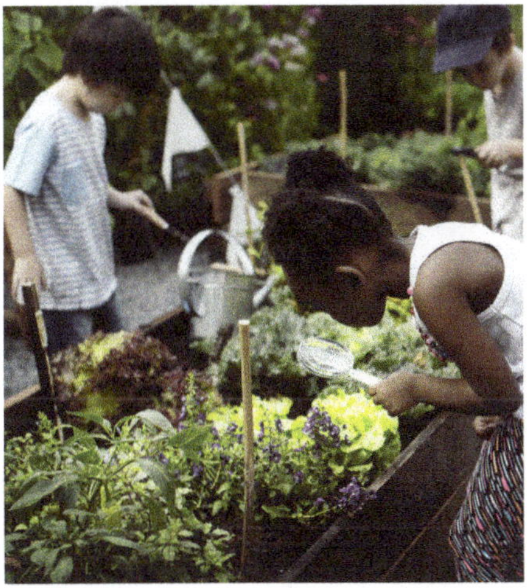

Another option if you have limitations with property, time or other constraints prohibiting your ability to create or participate in an outdoor garden, is to consider a tower garden. These are sold through many companies. The benefits include the ability to grow many items in a small space or a space with limited light exposure. They also include the convenience of timed watering and timed lighting with a large water basin that only needs to be filled weekly in many cases. These tower gardens can be used outside or inside. Their limitations include the inability to grow any root vegetables and the need to clean periodically, as well as cost.

In our family, we do utilize a tower garden, and it has been wonderful to grow various items year-round, such as basil, fennel, mint, thyme, dill, parsley, sage, chives, sorrel, cress, chard, collards, leaf lettuce, romaine, cabbage, beet microgreens and radish microgreens, and even catnip, as well as rosemary, lavender, spring-mix lettuce, kale, and vegetables such as tomatoes, beans and peas. (The veggies certainly take up a lot more space and are better when grown outdoors, in my opinion). It has been a blessing and a great way to teach the kids about growing our own food. They have been very receptive in broadening their food horizons with this. They love the fact that they can walk up and cut the lettuce themselves as we prepare their salad. Needless to say, salads have been a daily item on our dinner menu since the garden has been in place. And that's a great thing.

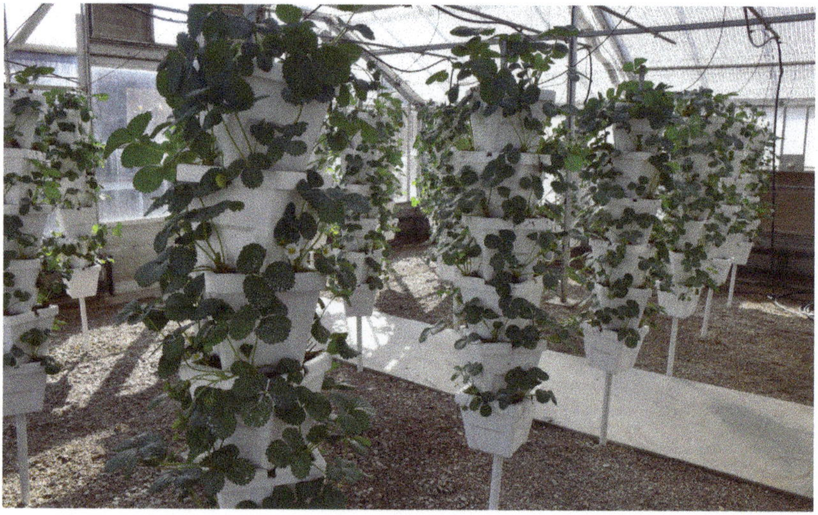

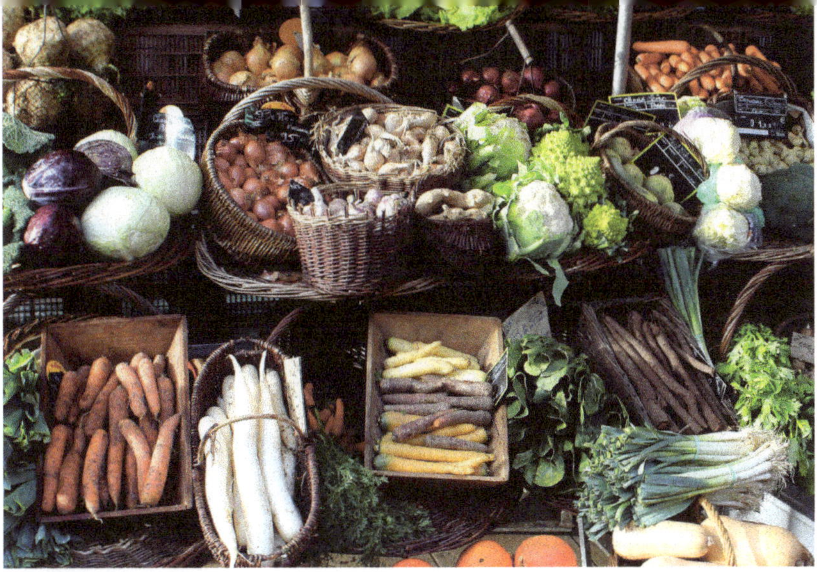

WHAT ABOUT:

ORGANIC FOODS

There are always questions that arise about the importance (or not) of organic foods. Chemicals are used regularly in non-organic food production, potentially at multiple stages in the process, which can be devastating to our health. These chemicals can remain in our food and environment, as well as our bodies, for decades. We do not fully understand the long-term effects that these additives could have on our health, because they are a relatively new addition to the human diet. However, some studies have found that they may have side effects such as headaches, nausea, weakness and difficulty breathing.

Generally, it is clear that certain foods are more laden with pesticides than others. Two reasons for this are insect popularity (insects are drawn to some fruits and vegetables more than others) and the fact that certain types of foods have more porous skin and thus are more susceptible to the potential absorption of chemicals than others. Organic foods do not utilize these chemicals. This is where the development of the "Dirty Dozen" and the "Clean 15" come in. These are lists to guide you if you want to be selective in what foods you purchase organic. With some foods, it is always best to choose organic, but with those less likely to contain pesticide residue, you can more safely choose non-organic. Updated every year, the Environmental Working Group's Shopper's Guide "Dirty Dozen/Clean 15" list is based on laboratory tests done by the U.S. Department of Agriculture Pesticide Testing Program. Note that if you buy any of the "Dirty Dozen" items non-organic - for example, apples - it is important that you wash them very well, or better yet peel them prior to eating, since they are more likely to contain pesticide residue. The "Clean 15" items are less of a concern regarding potential significant pesticide residue, and thus are considered to be safe non-organic choices.

Choosing organic products is more crucial for those who have weakened immune systems (those on immunosuppressant medications/chemotherapy), as well as young children and pregnant and nursing women. Studies with children who were fed conventional diets (non-organic) showed significantly higher levels of pesticide metabolites in their urine than in children who were fed organic food, and those who were changed from conventional to organic had their urinary concentration of the metabolites drop immediately to undetectable, according to the Center for Ecogenetics and Environmental Health. There are also concerns that chronic low levels of exposure to non-organic foods/higher pesticides in adults may be associated with respiratory problems, memory disorders, skin conditions, depression, miscarriage, birth defects, cancer, neurological conditions and ADHD.[27, 28] Certainly, these risks are highest among those with environmental occupational exposures, and this risk is less clear for the general population. From a *nutritional* standpoint of the food itself, there is no significant difference between organic vs. non-organic foods. They have the same vitamins, minerals, antioxidants, fiber, etc. The issue is purely one with a goal of avoiding chemicals and pesticides, since the use of these is unfortunately rampant in food production.

DIRTY DOZEN

Strawberries
Spinach
Nectarines
Apples
Grapes
Peaches
Cherries
Pears
Tomatoes
Celery
Potatoes
Sweet bell peppers

CLEAN 15

Avocados
Sweet corn
Pineapples
Cabbages
Onions
Sweet peas
Papayas
Asparagus
Mangoes
Eggplants
Honeydews
Kiwis
Cantaloupes
Cauliflower
Broccoli

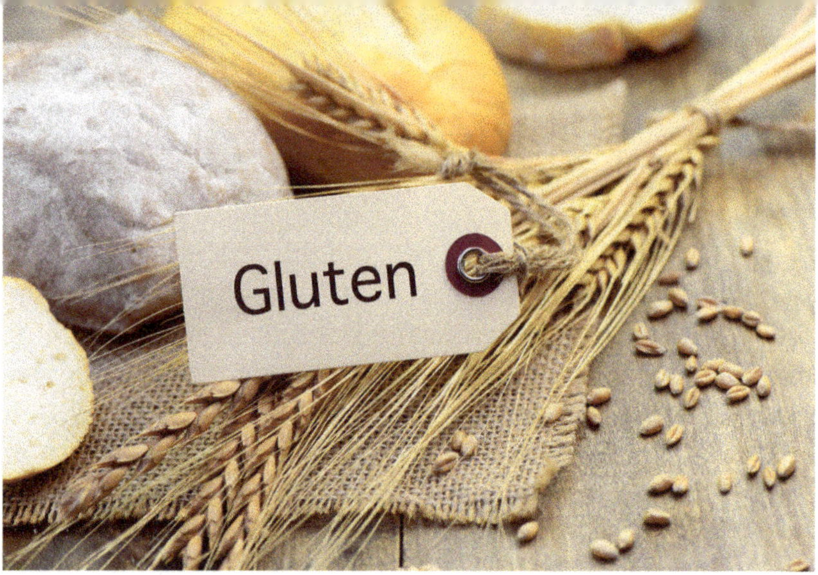

WHAT ABOUT:

GLUTEN

Gluten is a protein found in wheat, barley and rye. There has been a lot of publicity about gluten in recent years, and it has gotten a bad rap. While most people have no issues with it, certain individuals suffer from conditions for which gluten poses a very real problem. Celiac disease and gluten ataxia are rare conditions affecting less than 1 percent of the U.S. population. These are inflammatory immune system diseases that attack the body's intestinal lining and the cerebellar portion of the brain (involved in equilibrium), respectively. An additional rare gluten disease is true wheat allergy. These conditions require a lifelong gluten-free diet as the standard of care. There are antibody blood tests that can be done to support suspicion of the disease, but the true diagnosis for celiac disease is through a biopsy of the small intestine.

What most of the hype that the media is concerned with is NCGS, or *non-celiac gluten/wheat sensitivity*, which includes intestinal symptoms that improve once gluten-containing products are removed from the diet and after celiac disease and wheat allergy have been excluded. NCGS is quite common, affecting up to 13 percent of the U.S. population. Symptoms may include abdominal bloating and/or pain, diarrhea or constipation, headaches, fatigue, muscle and joint pains, brain fog and mood disorders, including depression and anxiety. NCGS has *not* been associated with an increased risk of autoimmune disorders, malabsorption or nutritional deficiencies. No laboratory or diagnostic test is available for this condition, therefore people who suspect this may be a problem for them need to do an *elimination diet*, in which they remove all gluten-containing items from their diet to see if their symptoms resolve. Typically we see that, upon reintroduction of those foods, their symptoms return. Many grains do not contain gluten, such as sorghum, quinoa, millet, oats, buckwheat (it's not really wheat), amaranth, teff, corn and rice.

Still, world trade in wheat is greater than all other crops combined. Wheat is globally the leading source of plant-based protein in human food, having a protein content of 13 percent, and when eaten as the whole grain, wheat is a source of multiple nutrients and dietary fiber. But it has been increasingly used specifically for the adhesive properties of gluten proteins used in processed foods, and this is what we would certainly like to avoid. Gluten proteins can be "hidden" in many foods including salad dressings, mayonnaise, soy sauce, BBQ sauce, gravies, soups, frozen foods (including french fries), processed cheese, potato chips, snack and energy bars, and a host of other unsuspecting items.

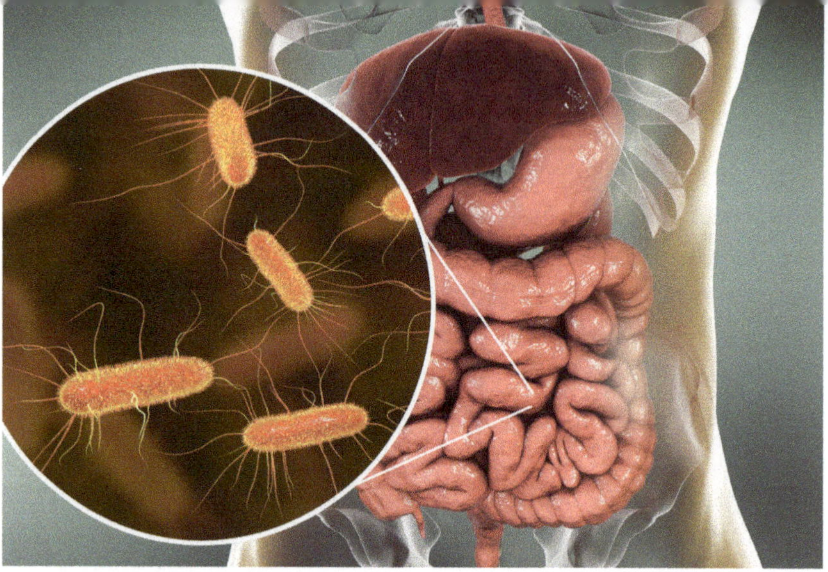

WHAT ABOUT:

PROBIOTICS AND OUR MICROBIOME

The term probiotic is derived from *pro* and *biota,* meaning "for life" in Latin. More and more evidence is mounting in support of consumption of foods and possibly supplements containing these beneficial live bacteria. Potential benefits have been demonstrated in the treatment and or prevention of several medical conditions: infectious and antibiotic- associated diarrhea, irritable bowel syndrome, chronic constipation, ulcerative colitis, Crohn's disease, Helicobacter pylori (ulcer-causing bacterial infection of the stomach), vaginal infections, urinary tract infections, Clostridium difficile (infectious) colitis, and allergies/eczema in children.

Foods containing live active probiotics:

- Yogurt (dairy or non-dairy), preferably organic and grass-fed if animal milk-based; be sure to watch the sugar content
- Kefir (cow, goat or sheep milk or water drink), preferably organic and grass-fed if milk); be sure to watch the sugar content
- Cheese (raw, not pasteurized, aged 6 months or more), including goat milk, sheep milk and A2 cow soft cheeses (many other cheeses do not contain live active probiotics)
- Cultured buttermilk
- Miso (traditional Japanese soybean paste)
- Fresh-brined refrigerated pickled cucumbers or other vegetables (many pickles do not contain live active probiotics)
- Kimchi (traditional Korean dish of fermented cabbage and vegetables)
- Sauerkraut (German, Russian, Polish and Chinese sour cabbage); look for the word "fermented" on the label
- Kombucha (fermented black tea)
- Tempeh (Indonesian soy product, often used as a meat replacement)
- Natto (traditional Japanese fermented soybean food)
- Cured olives
- Raw apple cider vinegar with "the mother" (this is fermented with probiotics, but most vinegars are not)

Of note, not all fermented foods have live active probiotic cultures. Beer, wine, chocolate, soy sauce and sourdough bread are just a few examples. Different strains of probiotics have different effects on the body, and it is becoming evident that having a variety of strains of these bacteria is preferred. It is difficult, however, to clearly recommend specific probiotic dietary supplements at this time, because in the U.S., they do not undergo the testing and approval process that prescription drugs do. It is unclear which strains and at what dosages deliver the best results. But overall, probiotics are generally considered safe.

Consuming a variety of fresh produce helps to maintain and protect your own microbiome, which is the 100 trillion microorganisms of over 500 different species that populate every normal person's healthy bowel, skin and mucous membranes (eyes, nose, mouth and genitals). These healthy bacteria keep pathogens (bad bacteria) at bay, as well as assisting in digestion and nutrient absorption, and are very much involved in our immune system.

Health conditions involved with our microbiome:

- Acne
- Asthma/allergies
- Arteriosclerosis (including heart disease)
- Autism
- Autoimmune diseases
- Cancer
- Dental cavities

- Depression and anxiety
- Diabetes
- Diarrhea
- Eczema
- Gastric (stomach) ulcers
- Inflammatory bowel diseases
- Malnutrition
- Obesity

The National Institutes of Health Common Fund-supported integrative Human Microbiome Project (HMP) was established in 2008 with the mission of generating research resources enabling comprehensive characterization of the human microbiota and analysis of their role in human health and disease. The information generated by the HMP is made available worldwide for use by investigators and others in efforts to understand and improve human health. Three current projects are focusing on pregnancy and preterm birth, the onset of inflammatory bowel disease, and the onset of type 2 diabetes. This is an exciting area of research with hopes for advancements in prevention and novel treatments of many chronic diseases. Stay tuned. In the meantime, feed your microbiome with a wide variety of plant-based foods.[29, 30, 31, 32, 33, 34, 35, 36, 37, 38, 39, 40, 41]

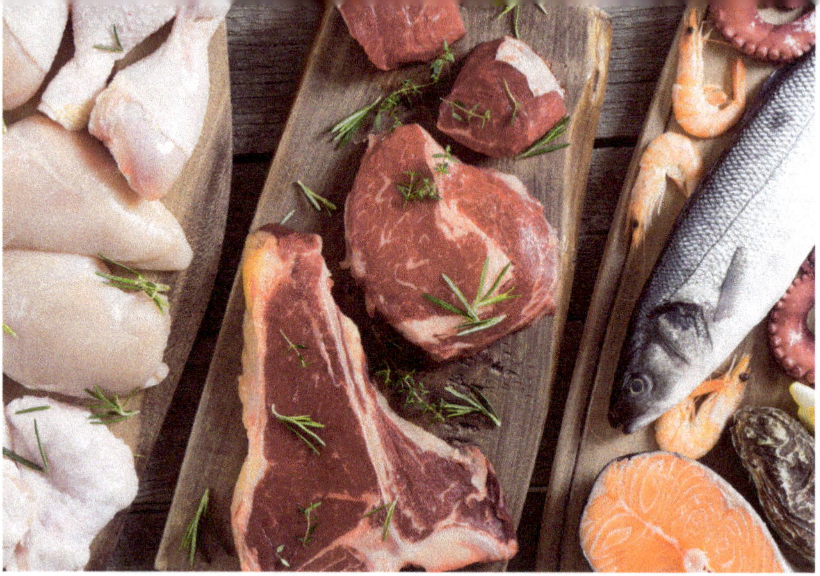

WHAT ABOUT:

MEAT AND FISH

The most important step to take with regard to meat intake is to decrease your family's intake of processed nitrite-containing meats such as bacon, delicatessen meats, hot dogs and sausage. A group of 22 experts from ten countries convened by the World Health Organization categorized that type of meat as "carcinogenic to humans."[42] (Carcinogenic means cancer-causing). When you do eat meat, stick to small amounts and choose leaner cuts such as pork tenderloin and top sirloin steak. The next most important step is to know where you are getting your meat from - literally. Choosing meat from a local farmer with grass-fed, free-range beef is far better for your health, your safety, the environment and the animal itself. The same is true for poultry. And hunting for your own meat is a good option as well.

Grilling meat over high heat produces cancer-causing amines and hydrocarbons formed by the charring of animal fats, while marinating meats and slow-cooking them (e.g as with BBQ) lessens the development of these dangerous substances. Grilling vegetables or fruits is not harmful, whether marinated or not, or cooked slowly or not.

Many animals are raised in unhealthy environments. This is the case with many CAFOs (confined animal feeding operations) run by large corporations. These conditions promote the rapid spread of diseases and thus the animals are at times treated with prophylactic antibiotics (given in an attempt to prevent disease). This widespread use of antibiotics with animals (and humans) has contributed to the rise of resistant bacterial infections. This affects people at every stage of life, including those most susceptible - infants, the elderly and those whose immune systems are compromised through chronic disease, medications or tobacco use.

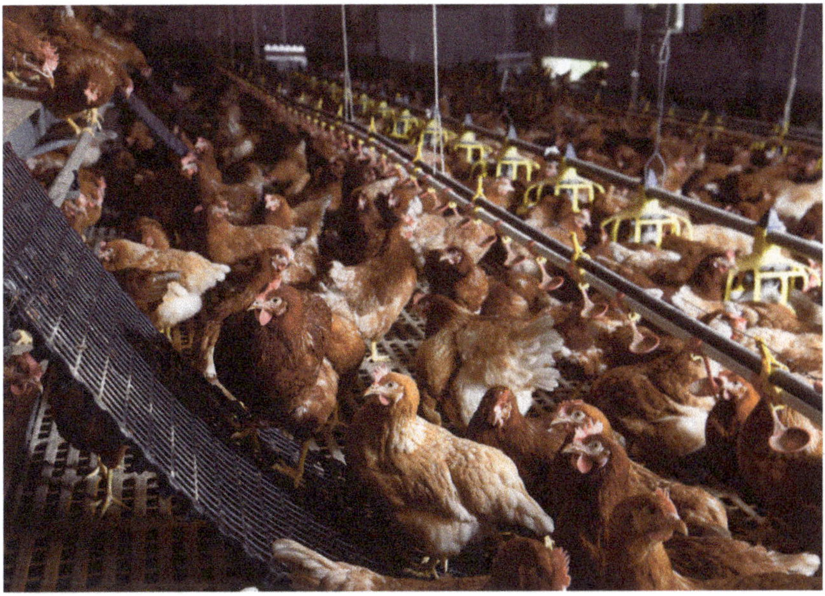

The confined animals are also often overfed with a diet of government-subsidized corn. Such practices decrease the quality of the meat produced and raise ethical concerns. The documentary Food, Inc. by filmmaker Robert Kenner, delves into this concept of socialized agriculture and its effects. It is worth viewing, but not with your children, due to some disturbing images.[43]

Fatty fish such as salmon are high in inflammation-reducing omega-3 fatty acids. However, significant and valid concerns exist about not only potential infectious risks of seafood, but also neurotoxicity due to mercury, as reported by the Environmental Protection Agency (EPA) and Federal Department of Agriculture (FDA).[44, 52]

Exposure to mercury most commonly occurs when people eat fish and shellfish that have high levels of methylmercury in their tissues. Almost all people have small amounts of this substance in their bodies, which reflects its widespread presence in the environment. Possible symptoms of mercury poisoning may include:

- loss of vision, especially peripheral
- "pins and needles" sensation, usually in the hands, feet, and around the mouth
- a lack of coordination of movements
- impaired speech, hearing, walking and balance
- generalized muscle weakness

A fetus can be exposed to mercury during pregnancy when its mother eats fish and shellfish that contain methylmercury. This exposure can adversely affect the unborn baby's growing brain and nervous system. These systems in the fetus are more vulnerable to mercury than the brains and nervous systems of adults. Children who have been exposed to mercury during gestation (pregnancy) can have negative developmental impacts in one or more of the following areas:

- cognitive abilities
- memory
- attention span
- language development
- fine motor skills
- visual spatial skills

Mothers who are exposed to methylmercury while breastfeeding may also expose their infant children through their milk, therefore the same precautions exist.

To limit dangerous exposure to mercury, these are the recommended serving sizes of fish for various age groups when limiting fish intake to two times a week from the "best choices" category, according to the "EPA-FDA Fish Advice":

- Age 2: 1 ounce per serving
- Age 6: 2 ounces per serving
- Age 9: 3 ounces per serving
- Age 11 and up: 4 ounces per serving

Fish are sorted into risk categories, with the "best" being the following species: whitefish, whiting, freshwater trout, tilapia, squid, smelt, shrimp, scallops, sardines, perch, pickerel, pollock, oyster, lobster, haddock, herring, crab, cod, clam, crawfish, catfish and butterfish.

Those considered to be the "worst" include king mackerel, marlin, orange roughy, shark, swordfish, Gulf of Mexico tilefish and bigeye tuna. You can visit the website for a complete listing by looking up "EPA-FDA Fish Advice: Technical Information."[44]

Another important thing to consider when choosing fish is farmed vs. wild-caught. The Cleveland Clinic, a world-renowned medical and research center, has an article posted on its website called "Fish Faceoff: Wild Salmon vs. Farmed Salmon," which was published in the journal *Nutrition* in 2014.[45] This article provides several important factors to consider when making your choice. One is that farmed salmon has over 20 percent more saturated fat, according to the USDA food composition database. This added fat comes with added calories as well, making wild-caught the better option from a nutritional aspect.

Next is the disturbing fact that persistent organic pollutants (POPs) are present in farmed fish ten times more than in wild-caught fish. These POPs have been associated with an independent increased risk of diabetes, obesity and other diseases, further supporting the preference of wild-caught fish.

Quantities of unsafe contaminants and cancer-causing chemicals are above what the Environmental Protection Agency (EPA) considers safe for frequent consumption especially in farmed salmon over wild-caught.

And lastly, the concern about antibiotic use has certainly been an issue in farmed fish in the past. It is currently unclear how much of this persists today, but it is not an issue with wild-caught fish.[46, 47]

With all the risks cited above with regard to consuming seafood, it makes one wonder what the benefits are. That would be the beneficial health effects of omega-3 fatty acids. But seafood is not the only way to consume omega-3s. Fortunately, there are several plant-based options as well, and as the theme goes with this book, it is preferred to get your omega-3 fatty acids from a variety of sources, rather than just one. And that is due to the variability of types of omega-3 that the foods contain, as well as other nutritional benefits that vary amongst these foods. Some plant-based foods containing omega-3s include: chia seeds, Brussels sprouts, algal oil (derived from algae), hemp seeds, walnuts, flax seeds, perilla oil (from perilla seeds, used most commonly in Korean cuisine) and grape leaves.

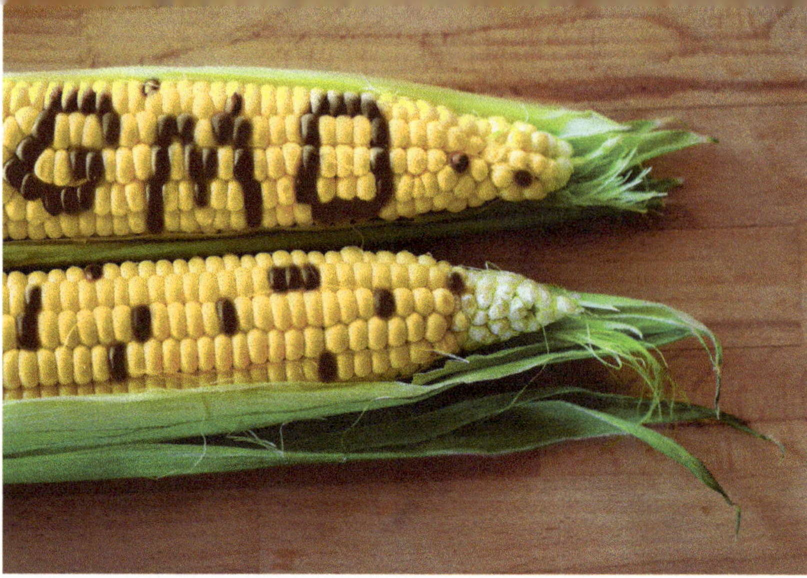

WHAT ABOUT:

GMOS

GMO stands for genetically modified organisms. GMF refers to genetically modified foods. Selecting and breeding of plants has been occurring for thousands of years; it has only been over the last few decades that the speed at which and the precise ability of this science has been able to occur through genetic modification. A benefit of this includes greater resistance to insect damage, increased immunity to plant diseases, as well as increased production of crops. In cotton plants alone, those genetically modified require much less chemical insecticide than do unmodified crops, leading to less pollution of air, water and soil. Between 1996-1998 alone, over 1 million gallons less chemical pesticides were used for growing cotton, according to the USDA. There has been a lot of publicity around this topic as well as misinformation on both sides - those who oppose and those who promote the use of GMOs. A major concern is the possibility of transgenic contamination. This is the contamination from cross breeding between a GMO plant into a non-GMO plant. Also concern for this transference of genomic material is potentially from ingested GMO foods into the commensal intestinal bacteria in human guts and subsequent transfer into human intestinal tissue. This is a theoretical concern, but one many individuals do not want to risk. However, to date there is no conclusive medical evidence to confirm their causality in cancer or chronic disease. According to Harvard University's publication *Signal to Noise Special Edition: GMOs and Our Food*, "The overwhelming majority of scientific evidence suggests that eating food with genetically modified DNA has no effect on human health, but there is also ample evidence that some GMOs have negative environmental impacts, such as the creation of superweeds." GMO crops far exceed those non modified in over 85 percent of soy and corn. Products made from these ingredients are vast including corn starch used in soups and sauces, corn syrup used in syrups and sweeteners, corn and canola oils used in most salad dressings, mayonnaise, baked goods and snacks. And so many more products- usually encountered when eating processed foods, condiments or eating out.

Eating fresh foods is certainly preferable to eating processed foods, and fresh GMFs are regularly eaten in vast quantities globally without any proven side effects. However, all manufactured foods with a long shelf life (canned foods, sodas, snack foods, and other preserved items) may have traces of substances that may contribute to or facilitate the development of cancer. Among the many compounds implicated include bisphenol A in the plastic linings of some metal cans, carbon dioxide gas in soda, and saccharin in sugar-free foods, in addition to those mentioned earlier in the discussion of processed meats. These molecules are not derived from GMFs. All effects are dose-related, and all are acknowledged to be cancer promoters in abusively high doses. [48, 49]

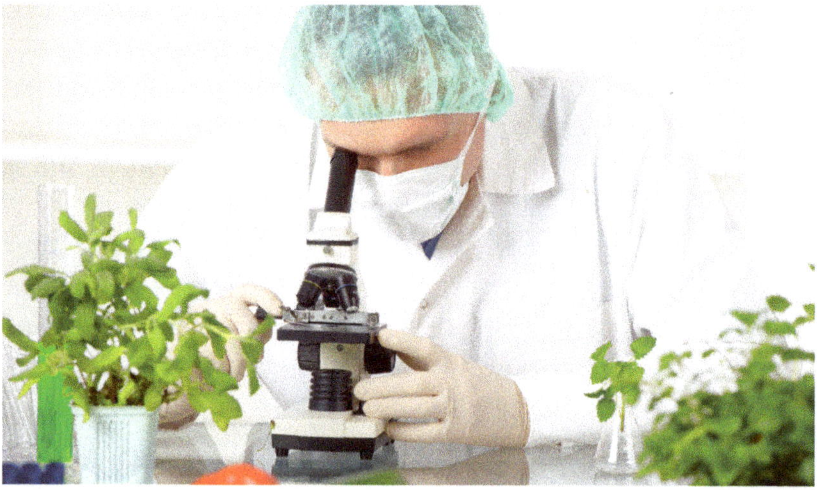

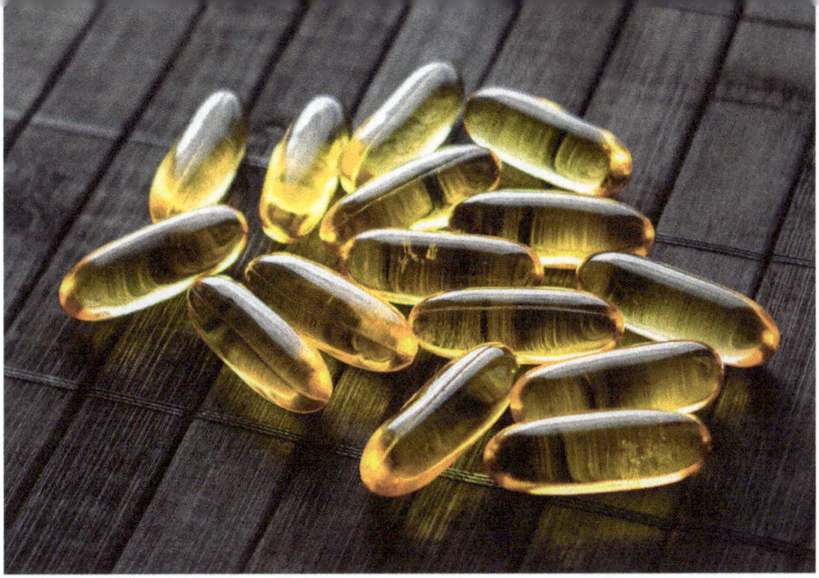

WHAT ABOUT:

SUPPLEMENTS

Many Americans use supplements, in part due to availability and extensive marketing. However, dietary supplements are regulated by the U.S. Food and Drug Administration (FDA) as foods, not as drugs. The label may claim certain health benefits. But unlike medicines, supplements can't claim to cure, treat or prevent a disease. The most popular nutrient supplements used are multivitamins, calcium and vitamins B, C and D, as well as fish oil. They may have benefits, but there are risks to be aware of as well.

According to the National Institute of Health (NIH), there is some evidence to suggest that calcium supports bone health, vitamin D helps the body absorb calcium, vitamins C and E are antioxidants, vitamin B12 supports nerve and blood cell health, and that fish oil has heart health benefits. Most people would agree that they have heard this before. Also that women often need additional iron and folic acid during pregnancy. But this does not mean that these nutrients must be obtained in the form of supplement. In fact, there may be risks to that. In 2016 a study published in the *Journal of the American Heart Association* (JAHA) questioned an increased risk of atherosclerosis (heart disease) in those taking calcium in supplement form. This is due to calcium deposits contained in these atherosclerotic plaques and the thought that the higher dose of calcium absorbed in a supplement form increased this risk. The same amount of calcium obtained through our food, however, did not show an increased risk, but rather a lower risk of heart disease.[50] When we get our vitamins and minerals through our food, they are absorbed more slowly, steadily and naturally. Not to mention that there are other immeasurable nutrients that often come along with the vitamins and minerals in whole foods.

Also of concern in supplement form is that fat soluble vitamins (A, D, E and K) can be toxic if taken in excess, as they are not readily excreted through our urine like water-soluble vitamins are. Supplements can also interact with prescription medications, so please notify your health care provider of any that you take. They may increase bleeding risk during or after surgery and can be particularly harmful in people with kidney or liver disease. Iron-containing vitamins can be fatal to children if taken in excess (e.g. chewable or gummy vitamins accidentally ingested because they were thought to be candy).

A study published in the *Journal of the American Medical Association* (JAMA) in 2014 showed a significant increased risk of prostate cancer in men who supplemented with vitamin

E.[51] Other known risks include Vitamin K which reduces the ability of some blood thinners to prevent blood from clotting. St. John's Wort can speed the breakdown of many prescription drugs (including antidepressants and birth control pills) and thereby reduce these medications' effectiveness. Antioxidant supplements, like vitamins C and E, might reduce the effectiveness of some types of cancer treatment. Many supplements are not studied in pregnant women or children, so be judicious with their use. Also be aware that many processed foods are enriched with vitamins and minerals, therefore in combination, the total daily intake may be even higher than one would realize for certain substances.

Certainly there has been some evidence of benefit with several supplements, including glucosamine (arthritis), turmeric (inflammation) and melatonin (sleep), among others, and most are generally considered safe in an otherwise healthy individual, but more studies are needed. To "fill in the gaps" nutritionally, especially with picky eaters, multivitamins can be used, but again are not routinely needed. Deficiencies are not very common and are mostly associated with people who do not have an adequate caloric intake (malnutrition), exhibit poor absorption through having chronic bowel disease or gastrointestinal surgery (especially bariatric weight-loss surgery) or have autoimmune conditions. Also, some medications can increase the loss of certain nutrients or interfere with the absorption of them in your small intestine. Alternatively, some supplements can reduce the absorption of prescription medication if taken at the same time, most notably thyroid medication. Therefore, be sure to discuss with your doctor or pharmacist not only what you are taking, but how and when you are taking these vitamins or supplements.

Although there is limited reliable data comparing synthetic multivitamins to whole food-derived supplements, there may be benefits to using one of the many brands of whole-food products available. Many are naturally processed from organic produce that is vine ripened and cold processed to prevent the destruction of the nutrients we spoke of earlier with regard to heating and cooking whole foods. These products also often contain cofactors and enzymes that may assist with the body's utilization of these nutrients and are of higher quality.

Questions also frequently arise about protein deficiency. We really don't see this in the U.S. in the absence of calorie malnutrition. If one is consuming an adequate calorie intake with a variety of whole foods, it shouldn't even be a thought. But, to look at it objectively, the average adult has a protein need of around 5 ounce equivalents (oz eq) *per day*, not *per meal* (as the USDA states) for adults, and 2-4 oz eq for most kids. As an example, 1 oz eq is a mere 1 tablespoon of peanut butter, ¼ cup of beans or ½ ounce of nuts! Often forgotten is the fact that whole grains have protein. It is when they are stripped of their nutrients from processing that they lose it. In fact, most Americans consume an excess of dietary protein, so one does not need to go out of their way, either with the added expense or the added calorie intake, to supplement with additional protein powders and drinks, especially those containing animal protein.[53] Spend your money on whole foods instead!

The FDA has established good manufacturing practices (GMPs) for dietary supplements to help ensure their identity, purity, strength and composition. These GMPs are designed to prevent the inclusion of the wrong ingredient, the addition of too much or too little of an ingredient, the possibility of contamination, and the improper packaging and labeling of a product. In addition, several independent organizations offer quality testing and allow products that pass these tests to display their seals of approval. These seals of approval do not *guarantee* that a product is safe or effective, however. Organizations that offer this quality testing include U.S. Pharmacopeia (USP), ConsumerLab.com, and NSF International (began as National Sanitation Foundation in 1944 and expanded to NSF International in 1990 to protect the world's food, water, consumer products and environment).

To make it easier to find reliable information, the National Institutes of Health (NIH) has fact sheets on dietary supplements at ods.od.nih.gov/factsheets/list-all/. NIH also launched an online Dietary Supplement Label Database at www.dsld.nlm.nih.gov. This free database lets you look up the ingredients of thousands of dietary supplements. It includes information from the label on dosage, health claims and cautions.[55]

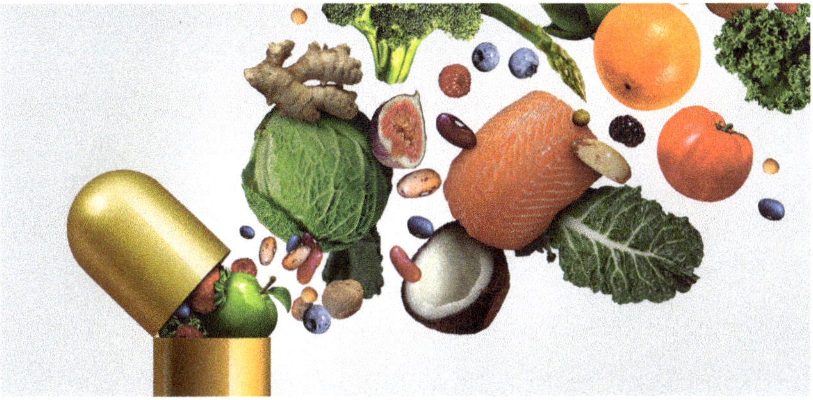

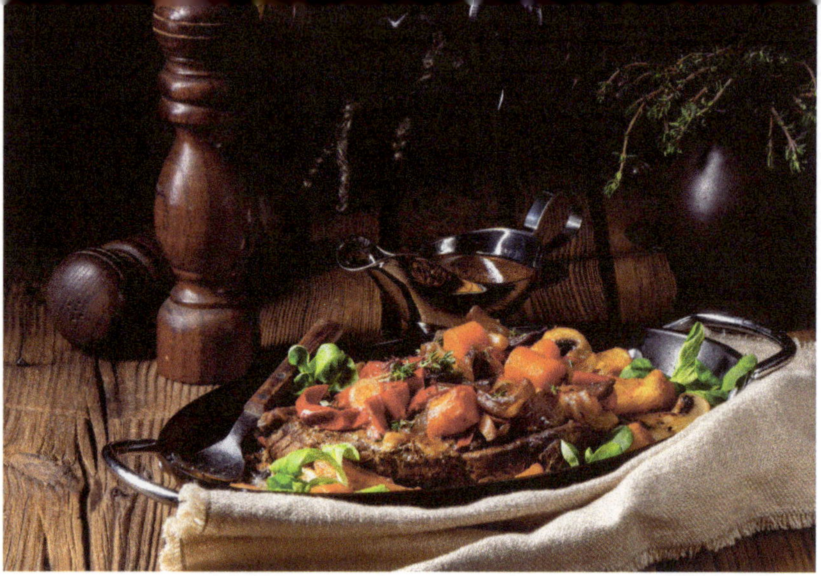

CONCLUSION

I sincerely hope that by reading this book, you have taken from it the message of "Vitamin V" as a goal to emphasize the incorporation of a variety of plant-based foods into your child's, your family's and your own diet. We are all continually trying to attain better health, and my aim with this book has been to present evidence to you that dietary changes incorporating an abundance of fresh produce may not only prevent or delay diseases such as heart disease and cancer, but in some cases may help to treat these diseases as well. Small changes can add up to big differences over time.

Reducing intake of processed foods and striving to prepare meals at home in the company of our families and friends reaps benefits that are immeasurable. Even if you were able to find only one way to incorporate "Vitamin V" into your shopping and cooking practices at this time, perhaps you could try again for additional ways in the future or research other ways on your own to do this. The evidence of the benefits in making such changes is insurmountable, coming from such reputable scientific organizations as the American Medical Association, the American Academy of Family Medicine, the American Academy of Pediatrics, Mayo Clinic, Harvard University, Cleveland Clinic, Oxford University, the National Institutes of Health, the World Health Organization, the Food and Agriculture Organization of the United Nations, the Federal Department of Agriculture, the U.S. Department of Health and Human Services, the Environmental Protection Agency, and the Physicians Committee for Social Responsibility, as well as many highly acclaimed medical journals and world-renowned physicians and scientists. All of these organizations, media and individuals, along with many others, are dedicated to promoting the health, environmental and cost benefits of transitioning towards more of a plant-based diet. These dietary changes can be liberating and exciting, opening up a world of new food experiences and traditions to pass on to future generations of your beloved family. Enjoy eating for health, and have fun with "Vitamin V!"

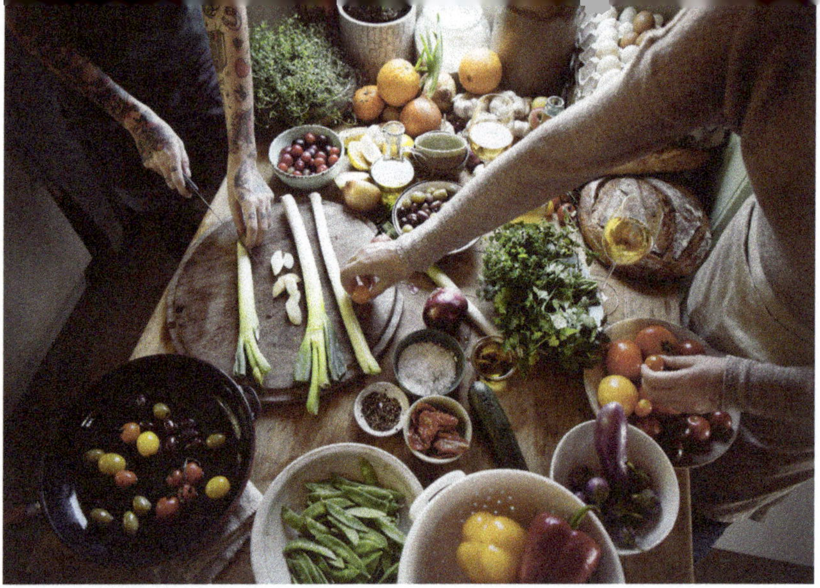

REFERENCES AND SUGGESTED ADDITIONAL RESOURCES

1. Heart disease facts and statistics, Center for Disease Control, https:www. cdc.gov and American Heart Association, https://heart.org

2. H. Kahleova, S. Levin, and N.D. Barnard, "Vegetarian Dietary Patterns and Cardiovascular Disease." *Progress in Cardiovascular Diseases,* May 2018

3. Emma J. Derbyshire, "Flexitarian Diets and Health: A Review of the Evidence-Based Literature." *Frontiers in Nutrition,* January 6, 2017

4. "Health Effects of Dietary Risks in 195 countries, 1990-2017: A Systematic Analysis for the Global Burden of Disease Study 2017." *The Lancet,* April 3, 2019

5. An Pan, Qi Sun, and Frank B, Hu, "Red Meat Consumption and Mortality: Results from Two Prospective Cohort Studies." *Archives of Internal Medicine*, April 9, 2012

6. Nikolas Scarmeas, Jose A. Luchsinger, and Yaakov Stern, "Mediterranean Diet and Alzheimer Disease Mortality." *Neurology*, September 11, 2007

7. Amy Locke, Jill Schneiderhand, and Suzanna M. Zick, "Diets for Health: Goals and Guidelines." *American Family Physician*, June 1, 2018

8. International Agency for Research on Cancer, Lyon, France, "Carcinogenicity of Consumption of Red and Processed Meat." *The Lancet Oncology*, October 26, 2015

9. Online health chat with Mladen Golubic, MD, PhD, "Benefits of Plant-Based Diets." my.clevelandclinic.org

10. H. Kahleova, S. Levin, and N.D. Barnard, "Vegetarian Dietary Patterns and Cardiovascular Disease." *Progress in Cardiovascular Diseases* May - June 2018

11. "Plates, Pyramids, Planet - Developments in National Healthy and Sustainable Dietary Guidelines: A State of Play Assessment." Food and Agriculture Organization of the United Nations and The Food Climate Research Network at the University of Oxford, 2016

12. Andrew Joyce, Sarah Dixon, Jude Comfort, and Jonathan Hallet, "Reducing the Environmental Impact of Dietary Choice: Perspectives from a Behavioural and Social Change Approach." *Journal of Environmental and Public Health, June 17,* 2012

13. Javier Mateo-Sagasta, Sara Marjani Zadeh, and Hugh

Turral, with contributions from Jacob Burke, "Water Pollution from Agriculture: A Global Review." Food and Agriculture Organization of the United Nations and the International Water Management Institute, 2017

14. "World Scientists' Warning to Humanity: A Second Notice." *Bioscience,* December 2017

15. Gene Stone, T. Colin Campbell, and Caldwell B. Esselsyn, *Forks Over Knives: The Plant-Based Way to Health/The How-To Companion to the Feature Documentary Forks Over Knives,* Turtleback Books, June 2011

16. Lauren Cassani Davis, "The Economic Case for Worldwide Vegetarianism." *The Atlantic.* March 28, 2016

17. Rosane Oliviera, "Cheap or Expensive? The REAL Truth About Plant-Based Diets." *UC Davis Integrative Medicine, March 3,* 2015

18. "The Importance of Family Dinners VII," a report from The National Center on Addiction and Substance Abuse at Columbia University, September 2011

19. William J. Doherty, "Share The Table: The State of Dinnertime in America." A white paper study on behalf of the Barilla Family Dinner Project

20. Marshall P. Duke, Robyn Fivush, Amber Lazarus, and Jennifer Bohanek, "Of Ketchup and Kin: Dinnertime Conversations as a Major Source of Family Knowledge, Family Adjustment, and Family Resilience." Working paper No. 26, Department of Psychology, Emory University, May 2003

21. C. Caffarelli, D. Di Mauro, C. Mastrorilli, P. Bottau, F. Cipriani, and G. Ricci, "Solid Food Introduction and the Development of Food Allergies." *Nutrients*, November 17, 2018

22. "Social and Environmental Impact of Palm Oil." *Wikipedia*

23. Prasanna Kumarathilaka, Saman Seneweera, Yong Sik Ok, Andrew Meharg, and Jochen Bundschuh, "Arsenic in Cooked Rice Foods: Assessing Health Risks and Mitigation Options." *Environmental International*, June 2019

24. "Arsenic in Your Food." *Consumer Reports*, November 2012

25. Justine Butler and Juliet Gellatley, "White Lies: A *Viva! Health* Report." Combining the findings of over 400 scientific papers from reputable peer-reviewed journals such as the *Lancet* and the *British Medical Journal*, http://www.vivahealth.org.uk, 2014

26. Sun Jianquin, Xu Leiming, Xia Lu, Gregory W. Yelland, Jiayi Ni, and Andrew J. Clarke, "Effects of Milk Containing Only A2 Beta Casein Versus Milk Containing Both A1 and A2 Beta Casein Proteins of G1 Physiology, Symptoms of Discomfort, and Cognitive Behavior of People with Self-Reported Intolerance to Traditional Cow's Milk." *Nutrition Journal*, April 2, 2016

27. "Health Risks of Pesticides in Food." The Center for Ecogenetics and Environmental Health, University of Washington, January 2013

28. "Toxic Chemicals in Our Food System." Factsheet from Physicians for Social Responsibility, 2014

29. Peter J. Turnbaugh, Ruth E. Ley, and Jeffrey I. Gordon, "The Human Microbiome Project: Exploring the Microbial Part of Ourselves in a Changing World." *Nature,* October 18, 2007

30. Fredrik Bäckhed, "99th Dahlem Conference on Infection, Inflammation and Chronic Inflammatory Disorders: The Normal Gut Microbiota in Health and Disease." *Clinical and Experimental Immunology,* April, 2010

31. H. Xu, H. Lu, "Acne, The Skin Microbiome and Antibiotic Treatment." *American Journal of Clinical Dermatology,* January 10, 2019

32. Andrea M. Kemter and Cathryn R. Nagler, "Influences on Allergic Mechanisms through Gut, Lung, and Skin Microbiome Exposures." *Journal of Clinical Investigation,* February 25, 2019

33. A. Fattorusso, L. Di Genova, GB Dell'Isola, E. Mencaroni, S. Esposito, "Autism Spectrum Disorders and the Gut Microbiota." *Nutrients,* February 28, 2019

34. Q. Zhu, R. Gao, Y. Zhang, D. Pan, Y. Zhu, X. Zhang, R. Yang, R. Jiang, Y. Xu, and H. Qin, "Dysbiosis Signatures of Gut Microbiota in Coronary Artery Disease." *Physiological Genomics* October 1, 2018

35. L. Sanchez-Alcoholado, D. Castellano-Castillo, L. Jördan-Martinez, I. Moreno-Indias, P. Cardila-Cruz, D. Elena, A.J. Muñoz-Garcia, M.I. Queipo Ortuño, M. Jimenez-Navarro, "Role of Gut Microbiota on Cardio-Metabolic Parameters and Immunity in Coronary Artery Disease Patients with and without Type-2 Diabetes Mellitus." *Frontiers in Microbiology,* October 5, 2017

36. S. Krishnaeddy, "The Microbiome in Celiac Disease." *Gastroenterolology Clinics of North America, March* 2019

37. M. Eslami, B. Yousefi, B. Kokhaei, M. Hemati, Z.R. Nejad, V. Arabkari, and A. Namdar, "Importance of Probiotics in the Prevention and Treatment of Colorectal Cancer." *Journal of Cellular Physiology, March* 2019

38. Shan Sun, Anju Lulla, MIchael Sioda, Karhryn Winglee,- Michael C. Wu, David R. Jacobs JR., James M. Shikany, Donald M. Lloyd-Jones, Lenore J. Launer, Andthony A. Fodor, and Katie A. Meyer, "Gut Microbiota Composition and Blood Pressure." *Hypertension*, March 25, 2019

39. C. Maldonado Galdeano, S. I. Cazorla, J.M. Lemme Dumit, E. Vélez, G. Perdigón, "Beneficial Effects of Probiotic Consumption on the Immune System." *Annals of Nutrition and Metabolism, January 23,* 2019

40. Ting-Ting Huang, Jian-Bo Lai, and Shao-Hua Hu, "Current Understanding of Gut Microbiota in Mood Disorders: An Update of Human Studies." *Frontiers in Genetics, February* 2019

41. G. Molina-Torres, M. Rodriguez-Arrastia, P. Roman, N. Sanchez-Labraca, and D. Cardona, "Stress and The Gut Microbiota-Brain Axis." *Behavioural Pharmacology, April* 2019

42. Véronique Bouvard, Kathryn Z. Guyton, Dana Loomis, Yann Grosse, "Carcinogenicity of Consumption of Red and Processed Meat." *The Lancet Oncology, October 26,* 2015

43. *Food, Inc.*, documentary film. Robert Kenner, director, 2008

44. EPA-FDA Fish Advice: Technical Information. U.S. Environmental Protection Agency, January 19, 2017

45. "Fish Faceoff: Wild Salmon vs. Farmed Salmon." *Nutrition*, March 3, 2014, cited in *Health Essentials*, http://www.health.clevelandclinic.org

46. J.G. Gormaz, J.P. Fry, M. Arazo, D.C. Love, "Public Health Perspectives on Aquaculture," *Current Environmental Health Reports*, July 15, 2014

47. Mercury Levels in Commercial Fish and Shellfish 1990-2012. U.S. Food and Drug Administration, October 25, 2017

48. L.Z.G. Touyz, "Genetically Modified Foods, Cancer and Diet: Myths and Reality." *Current Oncology, April* 2013

49. "Genetically Modified Organisms." *Nature,* 2000

50. J.J. Anderson, B. Kruska, J.A. Delaney, K. He, G.L. Burke, A. Alonso, D.E. Bild, M. Budoff, E.D. Michos, "Calcium Intake from Diet and Supplements and the Risk of Coronary Artery Calcification and its Progression Among Older Adults: 10-Year Follow-up of the Multi-Ethnic Study of Atherosclerosis (MESA)." *Journal of the American Heart Association,* October 11, 2016

51. Eric A. Klein, Ian M. Thompson Jr, and Laurence H. Baker"Vitamin E and the Risk of Prostate Cancer - Updated Results of the Selenium and Vitamin E Cancer Prevention Trial (SELECT)." *Journal of the American Medical Association,* October 12, 2011

52. U.S. Department of Health and Human Services, https://www.hhs.gov, Environmental Health and Toxicology,

https://www.envirotoxinfo.nlm.nih.gov, and National Institutes of Health, https:www.nih.gov. Websites for further reading, including resources on mercury, pesticides, lead and arsenic, among others

53. U.S. Department of Agriculture (USDA), Dietary Guidelines 2015-2020, Healthy U.S. Style Eating Pattern: Recommended Amounts of Food from Each Group at 12 Caloric Levels. Table A3-1, http://www.health.gov

54. *Overfed and Undernourished,* documentary film. Troy Jones, director, 2014

55. Dietary Supplement Label Database. National Institutes of Health, http://www.dsld.nlm.nih.gov.

56. Frank A. Oski, *Don't Drink Your Milk.* TEACH Services, Inc., publisher, 2013

CPSIA information can be obtained
at www.ICGtesting.com
Printed in the USA
JSHW021114291119
2643JS00014B/18

9 781950 659302